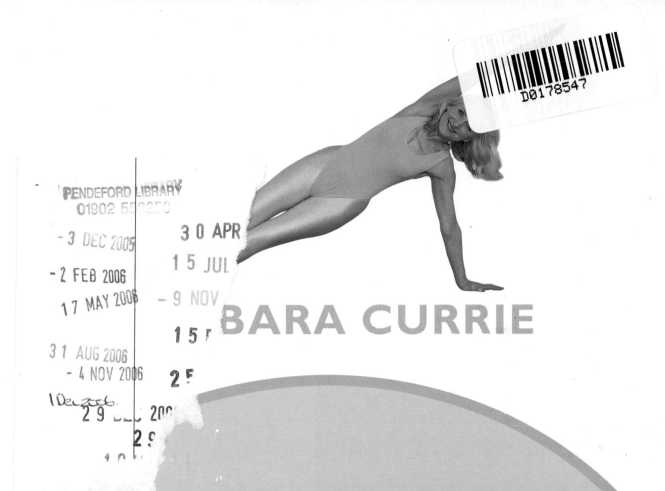

BARA CURRIE

# 10 MINUTES
## IN THE
# MORNING

## The 28-Day Yoga & Diet Plan

To my wonderful family: my husband Gordon, my children Lysanne and Mark, my daughter-in-law Rachel, my mother Babs and my brother Richard and his family, with my love and many thanks for your love, kindness and support.

Thorsons
An Imprint of HarperCollins*Publishers*
77–85 Fulham Palace Road
Hammersmith, London W6 8JB

The website address is: www.thorsonselement.com

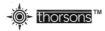

and *Thorsons* are trademarks of
HarperCollins*Publishers* Limited

First published 2004

10 9 8 7 6 5 4 3 2 1

Barbara Currie's website address is:
www.barbara-currie-yoga.com

A catalogue record for this book is
available from the British Library

ISBN 0 00 718955 9

Printed and bound in Italy by
Rotolito Lombarda, Pioltello, Milan

**Disclaimer:**
Not all diets and exercises are suitable for everyone. To reduce the risk
to you, please consult your doctor before beginning this exercise and diet
programme. It is designed for people in good health and is not suitable for
pregnant or lactating women. The instructions and advice presented are
not intended as a substitute for medical guidance. The writer and publishers of this book do not accept any responsibility for any injury or accident
as a result of following the exercise programme or for any health problems
experienced as a result of following this diet, or for any failure to lose
weight. The plan is followed entirely at the participant's own risk.

# Contents

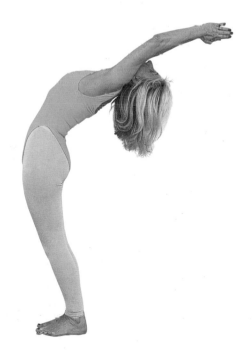

# Acknowledgements

I am most grateful to Belinda Budge and Wanda Whiteley for believing in me and making this book possible. Thank you Matthew Cory, Simon Gerratt and Nick Lake for your help, care and understanding while editing my script. Many thanks to Guy Hearn for the beautiful photography and to Sally-Ann Sexton for doing my hair and make-up for me with incredible care and patience.

Thank you to Polly Zabari for typing my initial script and making all the changes with a smile on your face.

Thank you Jacqui Caulton for the lovely design of this book, Sonia Dobie for the gorgeous cover and Kay Carroll for Production.

Thank you thank you to you all.

# Introduction

There is a time in every woman's life when she feels like taking herself in hand; she wants to lose weight, she knows she must exercise, she wants to feel better, have more energy, have more fun, look prettier and enjoy life more. She would like some great new clothes – but not until she has lost the weight that has been creeping up on her over the last few years. She would like to laugh more, have more self-confidence, but the main problem is *time*. Her life is already so busy she simply hasn't time to make special food or join an exercise class. Consequently, she feels depressed, frustrated, and out of control – and doesn't know where to turn.

Does this sound like you? If so, please cheer up, because that is why I have written this book. *10 Minutes in the Morning* entails a daily commitment of only 10 minutes a day for 28 days. These 10 minutes will be your most important minutes for the next 28 days. To help you on your way, this 28-day plan contains:

- Tips on visualizing and focusing on your goals;
- Uplifting and energizing quotes from some of the world's great motivators;
- Instructions on how to make your personal weight-loss planner;
- Daily menus containing easy-to-prepare, delicious meals;
- Daily exercises, for strengthening, toning and balancing your body;
- Beauty and lifestyle tips, to help you look and feel better all over.

By focusing daily on the weight you would like to achieve in 28 days time, and by visualizing yourself each day 10 lbs slimmer – and looking better for it – you will gradually become what you imagined. (To find out how this works, *see* pages viii–ix.) It is important to know that the world is how *we see it*. In order to feel healthy and positive, and achieve our goals, we need to uplift our spirits daily and concentrate on the good that is and always will be around us. To this end, for each day I have included some uplifting quotes that will help energize and motivate you.

The daily menus cover *everything* that you are allowed to eat and drink during that day. To help you keep to this, you will learn to make a weight-loss planner that you can always keep to hand. This will act as a reminder of exactly what you can eat – and the correct size portion – and the whole plan will fit in with your work, social and family life.

During the exercises, you will learn 3–4 yoga postures a day, 5 days a week, on Saturdays you will refresh your mind and body by doing the entire week's exercises, but on Sunday there will be no yoga – just a long walk in the fresh air. This means that at the end of your 28 days you will have learnt at least 60 yoga postures and have an exercise plan that will keep you fit and healthy for life! Don't worry if you think you are really stiff and inflexible at the moment, you'll be astonished how quickly you begin to improve!

Over these 28 days you are concentrating on *yourself* and achieving *all* your goals. And these goals might go a lot further than just becoming slimmer, healthier and full of energy – although that's a pretty good start! The beauty and lifestyle tips I have included will soon become a part of your life, helping to make you feel positive about yourself and look much better. And when you are feeling good about yourself, there is no limit to what you can achieve.

If you stick with my plan, at the end of your 28 days, you should:

- **Weigh 10 lbs less;**
- **Feel 10 times fitter.**

But, much more than this, you will have learnt:

- **The amazing life-enhancing power of visualization;**
- **Over 60 yoga exercises that will form the basis of an exercise regime to keep you fit, healthy and in great shape for life;**
- **A healthy eating plan to keep your weight off – for good!**

In short, you will have a comprehensive health-giving tool that is yours, not only for the next 28 days, but also *for the rest of your life*.

I bet you can't wait. Let's get started!

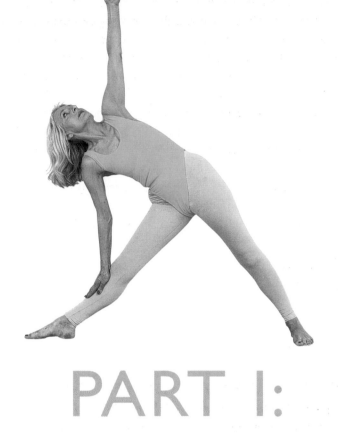

# PART I:

# MAKING THE 28-DAY PLAN

## Work for you

# The Amazing Power of Visualization

Most diets do not work for one major reason and that is that while they use vitamins, minerals, recipes and super foods they *never involve the subconscious mind*.

Your mind is the most important computer in your house, but while most people realize that their desktop computer needs programming, they give no attention to programming their own mind. Over the years, your mind will have been programmed by your parents, teachers, friends, aunties and uncles – and everybody else who has helped make you the person you are today. But along the way you were probably taught some extremely bad health habits. For example, if you were good you may have been rewarded with a bar of chocolate; if you fell down and hurt yourself, you may have been given a sweet 'to make it better'. And you may have been told you would never grow up big and strong if you didn't finish all the food on your plate. Twenty years later, probably you still reward yourself with chocolate or biscuits to cheer yourself up.

These are just small examples as to how our brains have been programmed regarding food. But more importantly, if you established a negative image of yourself in your childhood, you are probably still carrying that image around with you today. Maybe you felt unattractive and a big lump at school. If that is the case, it is likely you still see yourself as such and whenever you try to diet, your subconscious mind brings this image back to you, encouraging you to eat the amount it takes to keep you as an unattractive big lump.

But, *by changing the image you have of yourself, you can change yourself and be exactly as you wish*. This incredible power of the human brain means that you can re-programme your brain so that you *become exactly the weight and shape that you desire*. However, only you can do this for yourself. If you do not change your mental image of yourself, you will never lose weight or become the person you would like to be.

In his brilliant book, *The Power of Your Subconscious Mind*, Dr Joseph Murphy explains the power of the subconscious mind in this way:

*'There are two levels of your mind – the conscious or rational level and the subconscious or irrational level. You think with your conscious mind and whatever you habitually think sinks down into your subconscious mind, which creates according to the nature of your thought. The subconscious mind is the seat of your emotions and is the creative mind. If you think good, good will follow, if you think evil, evil will follow. This is the way your mind works.'*

This sounds so simple but it is so true. If you think of yourself as large and fat that is what you will become; no matter how few calories you try to consume during the day, your subconscious mind will make you grab that piece of cake or a snack to ensure you remain fat. Your conscious mind gives the command and your subconscious mind makes it happen. But if you tell yourself daily or, even better, 3 times a day, that you are beautiful, healthy, slim, agile and energetic, and *keep on* doing it, your subconscious mind will re-programme you to *make it happen*.

To assist you with reprogramming your subconscious mind, look through some magazines and find a picture of the body and shape you would love to have. Now buy yourself an attractive notebook and stick it on the front page. Next, find a picture of you smiling and looking good and stick your head on the picture of your ideal body, so that you can see how fabulous you will look.

Alongside this picture, write down your name and desired measurements; add to this a single sentence describing how you want to be, such as 'I am happy, attractive, slim and agile.' Make your own individual statement and be brave: think about the new ideal you and put it in your notebook.

**I am ...**
**My goal weight is ...**
**Hips goal size ...**
**Waist goal size ...**
**Thighs goal size ...**
**Bust goal size ...**

If you have another particular goal to achieve, such as a promotion, a salary rise or finding a new house, write this down as well in the present tense, for example 'I have got the promotion I have been aiming for and love my new job.' (Make it exciting, positive and happy.)

On the inside page write the date and the exact details of your weight and measurements before you start the plan.

**Weight ...**
**Hip size ...**
**Waist size ...**
**Thigh size ...**
**Bust size ...**

Now you won't need to weigh yourself again until Day 7, but focus 3 times a day on the positive image of your picture, your statement, your extra goal and your goal measurements and weight. Do this every day for the duration of the plan.

> *Imagination is the beginning of creation. You image what you desire; you will be what you imagine and at last you create what you will.*

GEORGE BERNARD SHAW

# The Diet

## Natural foods for health

Over 40 years ago, I began my training to be a state registered nurse at St Mary's Hospital, Paddington. I remember that while I felt very sorry for the patients, deep down I always wondered if anything could have been done to prevent their becoming so ill in the first place. At a later stage in my training, I moved to a ward specializing in nutritional and metabolism problems. One particular night, I was assisting the doctors with some tests on a patient and we became involved in an in-depth discussion on nutrition. One doctor suddenly said, 'If we all ate simple, natural food as fresh as possible, many of these problems and disorders could be eliminated.'

These words rang a bell in my brain – if a natural diet could help the patients, how about me? I had seen so much awful illness, I knew I wanted to stay well, and now here was a piece of information that was well worth trying. I started there and then, at the age of 19, to read everything I could find about diet and its relationship with health, and at the same time I focused my own diet on fresh natural foods.

I cut out all packaged and processed foods such as biscuits, sweets, cakes, chocolate, puddings, jams, jellies, pies and pastries; instead, I ate fresh vegetables and salads, fresh fruits and juices, nuts, eggs, cheese, grilled chicken and fish and fresh natural yoghurt. The results were incredible and I felt so well. I had much more energy, my skin was clearer and, although I have never been fat, I lost about 7 lbs in weight easily and without effort.

All the while I continued to read and learn. Most of all I wanted a beautiful slender body and *super health* – not gimmicks or quick fixes. I studied peoples such as the Hunzas who live in the Himalayan mountains and regularly are found working in the fields aged 100, frequently living to be 110 years old. I also read about the Okinawans who live off the coast of Japan and who are noted for their longevity. Both these have natural and fresh food diets and also benefit from mineral-rich water.

The thing that really made sense to me was to go back to our ancestors and discover what was the natural diet for mankind. Our Stone-Age ancestors lived on food that they could pick, trap or catch and studies show that their diet consisted of roots, berries, fruits, plant leaves, herbs, vegetables, a little honey (if they could find it), wild animals, birds, insects, reptiles and fish. Experts tell us that they ate most of their food raw. Scientific studies have shown us that Stone-Age man was tall and healthy with good teeth and strong bones. Today the isolated communities of the world who live on a natural diet of unrefined food are largely free from chronic diseases such as high blood pressure, heart disease, cancer, diabetes and arthritis. If we analyze the Stone-Age diet it turns out to be non-starchy and extremely low in carbohydrates, extremely high in vitamins and minerals, low in fat and high in protein and fibre. Whereas our modern Western diet is very high in carbohydrate and fat, low in vitamins and minerals and fibre and with a moderate amount of protein. Having read, researched and home-tested this fascinating subject I decided to make myself an eating plan to keep me in great shape and super healthy for life.

Our Paleolithic ancestors who lived some 40,000 years ago existed on a totally natural diet of fresh fruit and vegetables, leaves, roots, herbs, berries, birds eggs, animals, reptiles, insects and fish. Potatoes and bread did not exist, their soil was rich in minerals, they had no preservatives, additives or E numbers. Ready-made meals, sweets, cakes and biscuits were not available, food was eaten fresh or dried in the sun and in the main eaten raw. If they wanted to eat meat they had to catch it, find it or trap it. They had no idea what the RDA of their vitamins and nutrients were but experts tell us that they were very healthy, strong and muscular with no tooth decay and great bones. I think this is clearly the correct diet for mankind.

> ❝ *The further we, as humans, have moved away from the Paleolithic diet, the more susceptible we have become to Syndrome X\* and other diet-dependent diseases. In a very real sense, the best anti-Syndrome X diet is the Paleolithic diet – or at least a more modern and convenient variation of it.* ❞

JACK CHALLEM, BURTON BERKSON MD, MELISSA DIANE SMITH

I started my plan when I was 19 and although I gradually modified it as I continued to learn more about nutrition, now at the age of 62 it is still much the same as it was all those years ago. It has kept me very well, very flexible, feeling great and I am the same shape and weight now as I was then. I am delighted to be able to share it with you now.

**Caution:** Before starting this or any other eating plan I do recommend that you check with your doctor or nutritionist to make sure that it is entirely suitable to your dietary requirements.

# My Rules

## ① Do not eat between meals

This sounds incredibly simple but how life has changed in the last 40 years. When I grew up my mother used to tell me that it was bad manners to be seen eating in the street. Now people are mindlessly munching wherever you look and they have no idea of how much they really have eaten. If you add up all the snacks you eat during the day, you would probably be astonished at the number of calories you have consumed.

On my plan you will eat *three good meals a day and nothing in between* apart from a snack which you may have if your meal is to be delayed. By doing this you will train your body to be naturally hungry and at the prescribed mealtime.

## ② Never eat standing up

This is a follow on from the previous rule but is vitally important. Make yourself sit down and enjoy each and every mouthful of your food. By keeping to this rule you will cut out high-calorie snacks, quick nibbles and leftovers of the children's food – and the constant tasting of food as you prepare it. All these little snacks really can add up to a whole meal!

---

\* Syndrome X, or insulin resistance syndrome, is a name given to a host of diseases related to diet and insulin resistance – including obesity, heart disease, high blood pressure, high cholesterol, stroke, and a risk of cancer, depression and eyesight problems.

### ③ Eat slowly

Eat slowly and chew your food thoroughly. As well as helping your digestion, this also aids the function of your appetite controlling mechanism. If you eat too quickly, you can often feel unsatisfied by your meal and look to dessert to fill you up. If you eat slowly, you will eat less because you will put your knife and fork down before you have finished your meal. Always try to be the last to finish when dining with friends.

### ④ 'Only half fill your stomach with food, leave a quarter for water and a quarter for digestion.'

This wonderful ancient yoga saying is so important today. Basically, eat slowly and leave the table when you are satisfied but *never full*. This will leave you feeling light and energized after a meal but not full and bloated.

### Foods to enjoy

#### *Vegetables and salad ingredients*

All vegetables are allowed except potatoes, chips, crisps, sweet corn and baked beans, and all salad ingredients except pasta and croutons. Try to have as wide a variety as possible to achieve a balance of wonderful nutrients. Search out some lovely new salad ingredients and enjoy them, including:

| | | |
|---|---|---|
| asparagus | courgette | peas |
| aubergine | cucumber | pumpkin |
| bean sprouts | escarole | radicchio |
| beans (French) | fennel | radish |
| beetroot | globe artichoke | rocket |
| beetroot greens | kale | spinach |
| bok choi | kohlrabi | spring greens |
| broccoli | lambs lettuce | spring onion |
| Brussels sprouts | leek | squash |
| cabbage | lettuce (all types) | swede |
| carrot | mangetout peas | tomato |
| cauliflower | marrow | turnip |
| celeriac | mushroom | watercress |
| celery | onions | |
| chicory | parsnip | |

Have as much as you like of the salad ingredients – but only 1 tbsp of home-made salad dressing.

## Mixed Sprouts

Mixed sprouts are a wonderful addition to salads. These are easy to grow, delicious and highly nutritious, providing, weight for weight, more nutrients than virtually any other food. They are an excellent source of vitamin A, C and the B complex, fibre and protein. And they are so cheap – 1 packet, costing £1.99, keeps me in sprouts for a week! They are easily available at garden centres and health-food stores. I tend to buy mixed sprouts in packets which contain a lovely variety of delicious seeds. Some common sprouts are: alfalfa, fenugreek, peas, clover, broccoli, mung, and chick pea – but many more are available.

**Caution:** If you have lupus do not use alfalfa sprouts as they may trigger a reaction.

### How to Grow Sprouts

You need a jam jar, an elastic band and either a muslin cloth, a Jay cloth or similar. Put 1 tbsp of seeds into the jam jar and place the cloth over the top, fastening it into place. Half fill the jar with warm (not hot) water, gently shake the jar and then pour the water out without removing the cover. Place the jar on its side in a warm dark place. Repeat the process every day; on day 3 place the jar in the light. The sprouts will be ready to eat after about 4–5 days.

## Fruit

All fruits are allowed in the amounts shown in the daily menus. The best fruits for weight control are ogen and cantaloupe melons, raspberries and strawberries. Buy your fruits and vegetables in season and as fresh as possible. If possible, buy organic as they are free from chemical sprays and are grown in soils fertilised naturally.

| | | |
|---|---|---|
| apple | grape | pear |
| apricot | kiwi fruit | pineapple |
| banana | lemon | plum |
| bilberry | lime | raspberry |
| blackberry | mango | strawberry |
| blueberry | melons | tangerine |
| cherry | orange | watermelon |
| gooseberry | papaya | |
| grapefruit | peach | |

## Meat, fish and poultry

All fish, meat and poultry are allowed in the amounts shown in the daily menus.

| | | |
|---|---|---|
| bacon | ham | partridge |
| beef | kidney | pheasant |
| chicken | lamb | pork |
| duck | liver | turkey |

## Dairy produce and eggs

All cheese, butter, yoghurts and eggs are allowed in the amounts shown in the daily menus. You are allowed ½ pint semi-skimmed milk or soya milk per day. If you do not like milk, then you can substitute an extra 4 oz pot of natural yoghurt.

## Fish and shellfish (All fish are allowed in the amounts shown in the daily menus.)

| | | |
|---|---|---|
| bream | lobster | sea bass |
| calamari | mackerel | shrimp |
| clams | mussels | snapper |
| cockle | oyster | swordfish |
| cod | prawn | trout |
| crab | salmon | tuna |
| haddock | sardine | whelk |
| halibut | scallop | |

## Other foods

The following are allowed in the amounts shown in the daily menus.

- bread – only wholegrain
- mayonnaise – only home-made (see recipes) and strictly in the amount shown.
- nuts – all sorts in the amounts shown
- olive oil
- pasta – only wholegrain and only once a week maximum
- rice – only wholegrain and only once a week maximum
- salad dressings – only home-made (see recipes); no bought dressings are allowed
- walnut oil
- wine – one glass per day if desired

## Not allowed

- beers and spirits
- biscuits, cakes, sweets, pies, pastries
- bread – except pure wholegrain bread
- canned, dried or frozen fruits and vegetables – the only exception to this rule is tomato puree and organic tomato sauce and ketchup
- chocolate
- diet products – they may contain additives and preservatives
- fruit squashes and fizzy drinks
- hamburgers
- 'heat and serve' meals
- ice cream
- jams, jellies and preserves
- jelly and blancmange
- noodles
- packaged cereals apart from organic wholegrain ones
- pasta – except wholegrain
- pizza
- potatoes
- rice – except wholegrain
- sausages and made-up meat products
- sweet corn

Whatever you buy, think *fresh, fresh, fresh*.

## How much to eat

This is *incredibly important*. Food portions have grown tremendously in the last 20 years or so and with this has grown our ability to eat larger amounts than the body can cope with. So now you know the type of food to eat, it is vital to eat the correct quantities too.

I am sorry to say, I do not believe you can eat as much as you like of anything except for green salad leaves and then you must make do with just 1 tbsp of dressing.

### Fruits
**1 portion** =

- ½ of any of the following large fruits – grapefruit, papaya, mango, large banana, cantaloupe or ogen melon.
- 1 small slice watermelon or 1 large slice honeydew melon.
- 1 of the following – orange, apple, pear or peach.
- 3 of the following – dates, figs, plums, mandarins, kiwi fruit, apricots, slices of pineapple.
- 10 of the following – grapes, cherries.
- 1 small dish raspberries, blueberries, blackberries or strawberries.

### Vegetables
**1 portion** = 2 tbsp vegetables

### Salads
Have as much as you like, with the exception of avocados. Avocados are high in nutrients but are also high in calories, so I do not advise them in unlimited quantities. If you do choose to include half an avocado, then cut your meat, fish, eggs or cheese portion in half – instead of 4 oz prawns you would have 2 oz prawns and half an avocado with salad.

### Fish and meat
Try to have oily fish at least *3 times* a week and restrict beef, lamb and pork to 3–4 times a week.

## Liquids
### Water
*Try to drink at least 8 glasses of water per day*. Water is essential for our health as it hydrates our bodies and helps flush out the toxins. Most people do not drink nearly enough water, frequently confusing the body into thinking that it is hungry instead of thirsty. A glass of water will really revive you if you are feeling tired, so try to get used to drinking about 8 glasses per day. On a typical day your body loses water through exhalation, perspiration, elimination and urination, and if this is not replaced you can easily feel tired and dehydrated. In order to have 8 glasses per day, I keep a small bottle in my car and drink this on my way to and from work (when I am stationary!). I drink another small bottle while I teach my yoga

classes. I drink a glass with my lunch, when I am writing I keep a large bottle of water on my desk to sip through the day and then I have another 2 glasses at dinner.

Do try and do this. I promise you that not only will you feel much better, your skin will look much better as well. Think how a plant looks when it needs watering, it droops and its leaves look limp and wilted. Water it and see how it perks up – the same will happen to you!

### Tea

No more than 5 cups per day with ½ pint of skimmed milk from your allowance – decaffinated if possible. Have as much herbal tea as you like. An excellent tea can be made from 1 tsp fresh grated ginger in a mug of hot water.

Tea is an integral part of many of our lives so on your plan you are allowed *5 cups of tea*. Tea, especially green tea, does have a lot of health benefits due to the antioxidants known as catechins. Tea drinkers appear to have less atherosclerosis than non-tea drinkers and tea acts as an artery protector, an anti-coagulant and antiviral agent. Tea can make you feel slightly jittery so don't have it before bed or switch to a decaffeinated variety instead. I drink decaffeinated tea with organic soya milk.

### Coffee

Coffee can be great for people who wake up with morning lethargy. If you love coffee, remember no more than 2 cups per day – and *no tea*. I would make at least 1 of the cups decaffeinated. If you don't have tea or coffee with milk, then you may use your milk allowance either as a lovely warm drink before bed, or on your cereal. If you don't like milk have an extra natural yoghurt.

### Alcohol

Personally, I do not drink alcohol – it simply doesn't suit me – but I have allowed you one glass of either red or white wine per day. It can benefit your cardiovascular system. Red wine in particular can help ward off heart disease as grape skins are used in its preparation and these contain blood thinning agents, so enjoy – but no more than 1 glass per day. No beer or spirits. If you don't like wine, you may substitute a 4 oz glass of fresh fruit or vegetable juice instead.

## Supplements

If you are eating a good nutritious diet you should not need any supplements. However, our soils are not so rich in minerals as they used to be and we rarely know how long our food has been in storage. For this reason, I recommend that you take 1 good multivitamin and mineral tablet daily.

Finally: on a recent visit to a Brazilian eco-centre, our breakfast table held a sign which gives food for thought:

**Please do not feed the animals – an unnatural diet can make them fat, ill and aggressive.**

# Weight-loss Planner

Over the course of this 28-day plan, I have set out a varied and nutritious menu for each day. However, if you are unable to stick to this or want a little more choice, the following planner will help you choose.

## Breakfast

Choose from:

- 1 portion of fresh fruit and 1 × 4 oz natural organic yoghurt
- 2 portions of any fresh fruit
- 1 × 4 oz glass fresh fruit juice and 1 slice toast with a little butter and 2 oz cottage cheese or 1 boiled egg
- ½ grapefruit and 1 poached egg on 1 slice wholegrain toast and a little butter
- 1 × 4 oz glass fresh fruit juice, 2 rashers grilled bacon and 2 grilled tomatoes
- 1 smoothie (blend 1 banana, 1 natural yoghurt with 6 fresh strawberries or a small carton of raspberries)
- 2 egg omelette and 3 grilled mushrooms

## Lunch

Choose from:

- 4 oz fresh grilled chicken, turkey or fish (hot or cold)
- 4 oz red meat (remember red meat is only allowed 3–4 times per week)
- 6 oz cottage cheese or 2 oz hard cheese

and

- a large mixed salad from the list of ingredients (*see* page xii). Remember to try and vary them everyday. Enjoy this with 1 tbsp dressing. Instead of salad you may have 2 cooked vegetables.

or

- 1 sandwich made with 2 thin slices wholegrain bread with a scraping of butter or mayonnaise filled with salad and 2 oz chicken, turkey or fish or 1 oz cheese.

*Dessert* – 1 portion fresh fruit

## Dinner

- 4 oz chicken, fish, veal or red meat (red meat is only allowed 3–4 times per week)

or

- 1 small wholegrain rice or pasta dish (no more than twice per week)

and

- 2 fresh vegetables or a large salad with 1 tbsp dressing.

**Dessert** – 1 portion fresh fruit

## To drink

Eight glasses of water per day. Herbal tea as desired. No more than 5 cups of tea or 2 cups of coffee per day and semi-skimmed milk or soya milk from your allowance of ½ pint. If you do not like milk then have an extra 4 oz pot of natural yoghurt. 1 glass of wine is allowed per day if desired or 4 oz of fruit or vegetable juice.

This plan will fit in with your life no matter how busy you are – you have plenty of choice but remember *no more* than 4 oz of chicken, fish or red meat and *no snacks*. The only exception to this is if your meal is unavoidably delayed; in that case, instead of having 1 portion of fruit for your dessert, have it as a snack prior to your meal but do remember to sit down and eat it. If fruit is included in your lunch or dinner (for instance, chicken and mango salad) then you may not have an extra portion of fruit for dessert. If fruit is used as a garnish (for instance, pork and apple sauce), then have ½ a fruit portion for dessert. This may sound pedantic but it is the details that matter.

It will help if you carry the weight-loss planner with you until you become accustomed to it and to give you great meal choices at every restaurant or eating place you visit. You will be able to eat out anywhere and no one will ever know you are on a diet.

## In restaurants

Have a lovely salad as a starter and then your choice of chicken, fish or meat as a main course with 1 vegetable portion, and follow with fruit, such as a bowl of fresh raspberries.

# The Exercises

My constant search for super health led me to discover yoga over 30 years ago. It clicked with me immediately and felt just perfect. It has kept me in the same shape I was in my 20s, has given me energy, kept my spine and joints flexible and in great condition, and helped me to relax and sleep well. Much more than this, its profound teachings and techniques have helped me through life's many challenges.

## About yoga

The word yoga means the union of body, mind and spirit with the universal spirit. Its exact origins are unclear but it is thought to have been developed around 5000BC in an area of pre-historic India that is now part of Pakistan. Yoga combines thorough physical exercises, balancing postures and deep-breathing practices with meditation and deep relaxation.

The exercises work on literally 100 per cent of the body – toning, firming, sculpting and realigning it whilst toning it internally as well. The movements are performed carefully and slowly. They are particularly excellent for ridding the body of the tension which is so pervasive in our stressful modern world. Tension literally strangles our bodies, inhibiting both lymph and blood flow to our tissues. The blood system carries nutrients from the food we eat and oxygen from the air we inhale to our cells whilst the lymphatic system removes toxins and fights infection. It is easy to understand that if these systems are inhibited by chronic stress this can easily cause deterioration in our bodies. By carefully stretching away all tension and by deep breathing to stimulate oxygen to the tissues, yoga's soothing calming movements help restore these functions. The balancing movements strengthen our bodies and keep our joints flexible but they necessitate a huge level of concentration. By concentrating the mind while positioning the body, yoga ensures we stay in the present moment and takes the mind off its day-to-day concerns, thereby giving it a necessary rest. The breathing exercises are both calming and relaxing and once learnt can be used anywhere to help you unwind.

The mind is difficult to tame and the more frenetic our lives become the more we need yoga to help us calm down. Meditation and relaxation are wonderful tools to help us relax at will; eventually we realize the peace and happiness we seek is not out there but within ourselves and yoga is there to help us attain it.

## Practising yoga

Yoga can be fitted into the busiest life style. All you need to practice it is a warm airy room, loose clothing, bare feet and a mat or rug to sit on. Always wait about 2 hours after a main meal before practising yoga and make sure you won't be disturbed – make this your time.

Yoga is for everyone but *the golden rule is you must never strain*. Move carefully and slowly into each movement, hold it for the prescribed length of time and never worry if you are stiff and uncoordinated to start with. We are all stiff in the beginning but as you practice you will find yourself making rapid progress and looking and feeling much better into the bargain.

## Breathing

In yoga we breathe deeply with each movement to stimulate the body with life-giving oxygen. In general, gently push your abdominal muscles out and inhale slowly through your nose as you start to stretch into a posture. As you move into the movement slowly and calmly exhale through your nose. While relaxing in the movement just breathe normally and peacefully through your nose.

**Caution**: Although yoga is for all ages, it is for healthy people and if you have any health queries whatsoever then please check with your doctor before you start.

# Ten Minutes in the Morning 28-Day Plan

### *Before you begin:*

1 Find a notebook.
2 Paste in your beautiful body picture with your head on it.
3 Weigh yourself and enter your measurements into the book.
4 Enter your goal measurements into your notebook and make your daily affirmation or statement.
5 If you have another goal that you would like to achieve, enter this as well.
6 Check your food cupboards and buy enough fresh food for your first 3 days.
7 Give away anything that could be a temptation.
8 Set your alarm clock 10 minutes early for tomorrow morning.

## The magic formula

When you combine daily visualization with inspiration and daily action you can achieve any goal.

- Take 2 minutes: to read the quotation. Visualize your goals and be grateful for the blessings you already possess.
- Take 1 minute: to read through today's menu suggestions.
- Take 5 minutes: to exercise.
- Take 2 minutes: to read the beauty or lifestyle tip.

> ❛ *A good plan is like a road map. It shows the final destination and usually marks the best way to get there.* ❜
>
> H. STANLEY JUDD

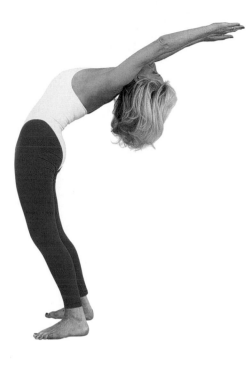

# PART II:

# THE
# 28-DAY PLAN

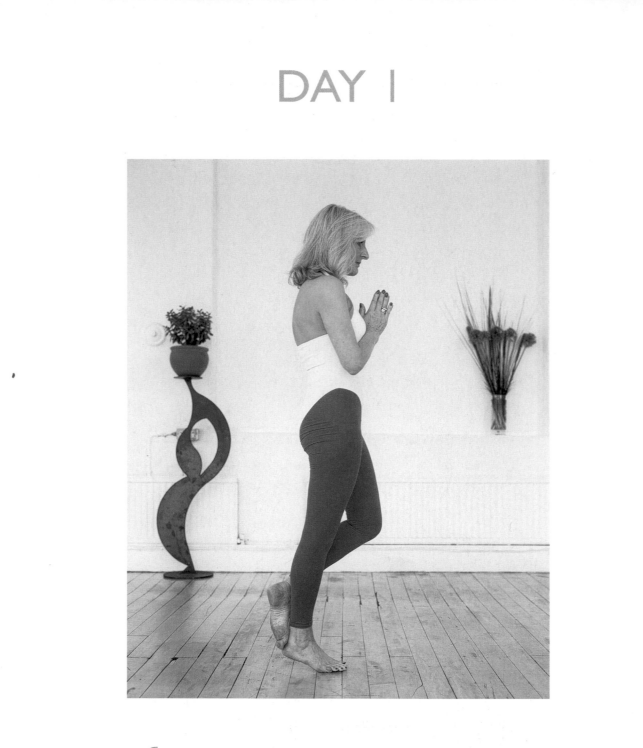

6 *To understand the magical nature of the mind
is to acquire awesome power. It is to understand that
at every moment of our lives we have the power to
accomplish anything we want.* 9

DEEPAK CHOPRA

## TAKE 2 MINUTES: to focus on your goals

Focus on your goals – look at your picture and visualize yourself having that beautiful firm polished body. Visualize your extra goal. If it is a promotion, visualize your new job and see yourself in this great new position. Review your day ahead, think in advance about any potential challenges and visualize yourself overcoming them with ease.

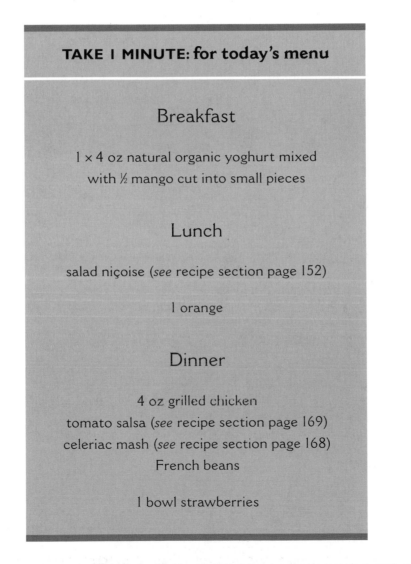

## TAKE 1 MINUTE: for today's menu

### Breakfast

1 x 4 oz natural organic yoghurt mixed
with ½ mango cut into small pieces

### Lunch

salad niçoise (*see* recipe section page 152)

1 orange

### Dinner

4 oz grilled chicken
tomato salsa (*see* recipe section page 169)
celeriac mash (*see* recipe section page 168)
French beans

1 bowl strawberries

**Daily Allowances:** please bear in mind that you can always have your daily allowance of 1 glass of wine or 4 oz fruit or vegetable juice; 5 cups of tea or 2 cups of coffee with milk (from your allowance of ½ pint semi-skimmed or soya milk); unlimited herbal tea and 8 glasses of water. This applies to every day of the plan.

# 1 Upward stretch forwards and backwards bend

This brilliant revitalizing morning stretch releases tension from the entire body, corrects posture and gives amazing flexibility to the spine. It slims and tones the abdomen, midriff, waistline and throat and firms and tones the backs of the thighs and calves. By encouraging blood flow to the head and neck area, it boosts the condition of the skin, hair and brain cells.

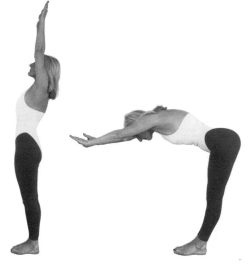
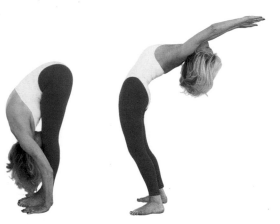

- Stand straight with your feet facing forwards and about 12 in apart. Correct your posture.
- Inhale and lift your arms straight up above your head.
- Exhale slowly as you move forwards keeping your back flat and your legs straight. Don't strain.
- Relax in your maximum position and hold the movement for a count of 5, breathing normally.
- Your eventual aim is to have your hands flat on the floor and your chin on your shins.
- Inhale and lift your head first, then slowly, keeping your back flat and legs straight, return to an upright position.
- Stretch your arms up above your head, then without straining, and keeping your eyes on your thumbs, slowly relax backwards exhaling in your maximum position. Hold for a count of 5.
- Your eventual aim is a beautiful backwards arch as shown.
- Inhale as you slowly return to an upright position.
- Exhale, lower your arms and relax.
- Repeat twice.

### Extra Help

*It is not until we start to work the spine that we realize just how stiff we have become. I know, I have been there! The body operates on a 'use it or lose it' system but even if initially you are really stiff, with daily practice even the stiffest back can regain its youthful flexibility. Remember not to strain, relax in your own maximum position even if you can move very little in the beginning, and you will be delighted at how quickly your flexibility improves and how much better you feel.*

*Moving backwards for the first time can present a huge challenge, but keep your eyes on your thumbs, relax and even if you only move back an inch in the beginning stages, with practice this will improve very quickly, I promise.*

# 2 Sideways stretch

This movement is great for slimming and toning the midriff and waistline, giving the spine tremendous flexibility and releasing tension in the lower back.

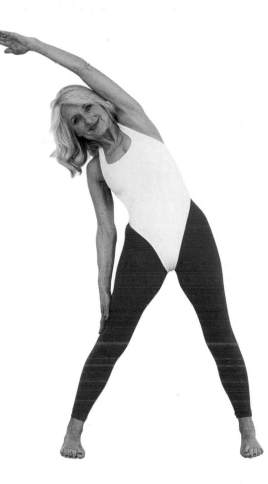

- Stand straight with your feet facing forwards and about 3 ft apart.
- Breathe in and lift your left hand in the air.
- Exhale and keeping your body in line, slide your right hand down your right leg as far as possible. Keep your left arm straight and have the inner part of the left arm by your left ear.

- Hold your maximum stretch for a count of 5.
- Inhale and slowly and smoothly return to an upright position.
- Exhale, slowly lower your arm and relax.
- Repeat the movement on the other side and then repeat the entire sequence twice.

### Extra Help
*There is a huge temptation to bend forwards in this movement to get your hand further down the leg. Please don't. Keep your body straight and look forwards. The slow careful movement is excellent for toning and slimming your midriff and waistline.*

# 3   Rishi's posture

This movement is brilliant for releasing deep-seated tension and rebalancing the lower back. I really recommend it for people with lop-sided jobs (such as a dentist) or people who play imbalanced sports such as tennis or golf. Gardeners can also find it really helpful to release the tension resulting from being in awkward positions for a considerable length of time. It will tone and firm your midriff, waistline, bottom and thighs and keep your back in great condition enhancing its flexibility. It relieves tension from the chest and firms your jaw and throat.

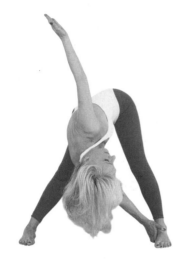

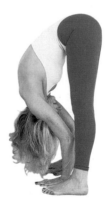

- Stand straight with perfect posture, your feet 3 ft apart with your toes facing forwards not outwards.
- Lift your arms straight up in the air as you inhale.
- As you exhale with your back flat and legs straight, move forwards to your own maximum position without strain.
- Slide your right hand to your left leg, grabbing it wherever it is comfortable, but don't bend your knees. Eventually your aim is to place your right hand under your left foot.
- Lift your left arm in the air; now slowly and carefully turn your body so that you are looking at your left hand.

- Hold this position for a count of 5, breathing normally, then slowly lower your arm and relax forwards.
- Now repeat to the other side, sliding the left hand on to your maximum position on your right leg and lifting your right arm in the air. Hold for a count of 5 then slowly lower your arm and let your body relax in its maximum forwards bend. Hold this position for a count of 5, breathing normally.
- Grab your legs and gently, keeping your back straight, draw your body inwards towards your legs.

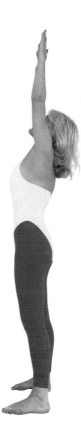

- Inhale deeply and lift your head, then slowly return to an upright position and stretch your arms up above your head.
- Now place your hands at your waistline with your thumbs in front and fingers behind. Inhale deeply and with a full lung; bend

backwards exhaling in your maximum backwards bend for a count of 5, breathing normally.
- Inhale gently as you return to an upright position.
- Exhale, relax and repeat the entire sequence.

## TAKE 2 MINUTES: beauty tip

*May no one ever come to you without going away better and happier. Everyone should see kindness in your face, in your eyes, in your smile.*

MOTHER TERESA

Today let everyone see your smile – it will make both of you feel better.

# DAY 2

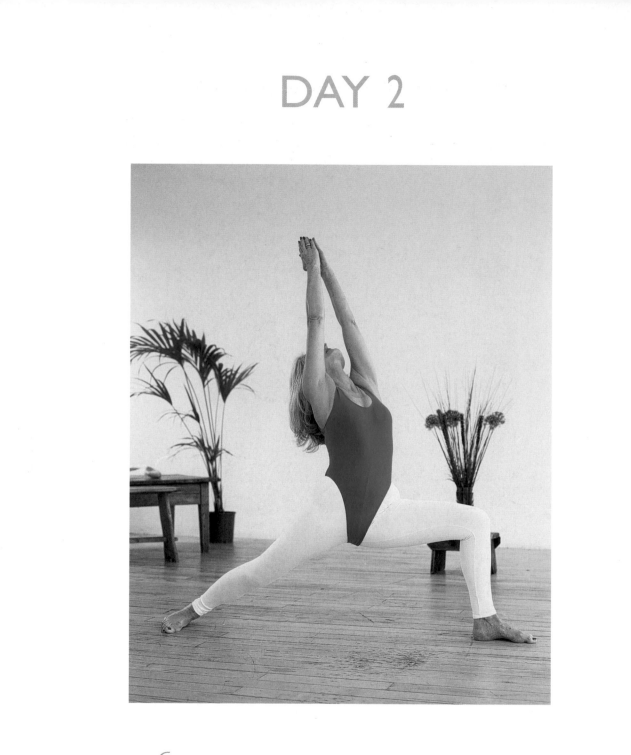

*If one advances confidently in the direction of his dreams and endeavours to live the life which he has imaged, he will meet with success unexpected in common hours.*

HENRY DAVID THOREAU

## TAKE 2 MINUTES: to focus on your goals

Look in your notebook, visualize your goal – see yourself beautifully toned and slim. Take a minute to visualize yourself like this, focusing also on your achievement goals. Focus on having a really great day. Visualize great meetings and lovely new opportunities.

## TAKE 1 MINUTE: for today's menu

### Breakfast

½ mango with blueberries
and a squeeze of lime

### Lunch

chicken and papaya salad (*see* recipe page 152)

### Dinner

4 oz grilled salmon with pesto (*see* recipe page 170),
steamed broccoli and mashed squash

½ cantaloupe melon

# 1  Chest expansion

On the physical level, this movement is amazing in how it tones your upper arms and releases the tension in the back of your neck and shoulders. In the forward bend it will tone the back of your thighs and calves and stimulate blood flow to the head and neck area so benefiting your skin, hair and brain cells. While bending backwards it frees the chest of tension and firms the jaw and throat.

The tensions of the mind are frequently stored in the back of the neck (the proverbial pain in the neck) and lumbar spine – this powerful movement carefully helps both these areas. This movement is one of my pupils' favourite positions. It is excellent for removing tension from the neck and shoulders. It also stimulates blood flow to the head and neck area and helps to revive a dull skin and lacklustre hair. When we do the movement in class a real sigh of relief echoes around the room as dormant tensions are released.

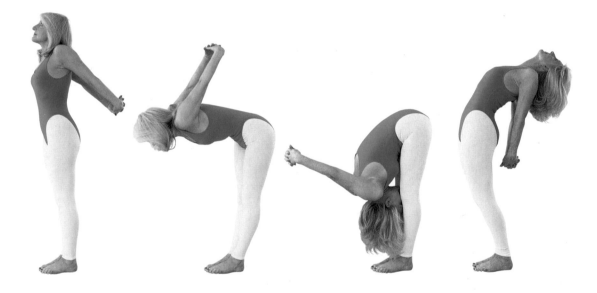

- Stand with your feet together and your back absolutely straight. Interlock your hands behind your back and gently pull your shoulders back, straightening your arms.
- Inhale and lift your arms up as high as possible behind your back, then exhale as you slowly bend forwards with flat back and straight legs into your maximum forwards bend. Relax in your maximum position and breathe normally in it and hold the position for a count of 5. Eventually your aim is to place your chin on the top of the shin just under the knee. It will happen, but remember not to strain!

- Inhale and lift your head first, then slowly return to an upright position and gently bend backwards pulling your arms back down and under your bottom. Exhale in your maximum position and hold for a count of 5, breathing normally.
- Inhale and return to an upright position, hold your arms up behind your back for an extra count of 2, then lower them and relax.
- Repeat twice.

# 2   Siamese posture

This movement does wonders for your waistline and midriff, keeps your spine flexible and tones your throat and jaw.

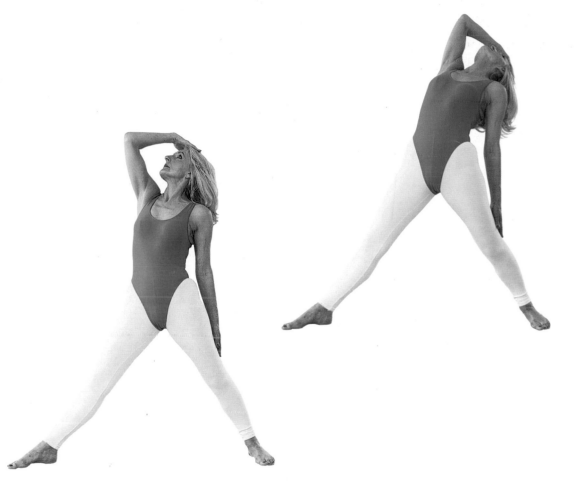

- Stand straight with your legs 3½–4 ft apart.
- Turn your right foot at a 90° angle to the right.
- Place your right hand on the top of your head and look at the centre of your elbow.
- Inhale deeply, then as you exhale slide your left hand down your left leg as far as

possible. Keep your gaze on the centre of your elbow.
- Hold your maximum stretch for a count of 5, breathing normally, then inhale and return to an upright position, exhale and relax and repeat on the left side then repeat the entire sequence.

# 3   Warrior posture

## STAGE 1

The warrior posture firms and tones your thighs and releases lower back tension. It gives fantastic shape to your legs streamlining your calves and firming your buttocks.

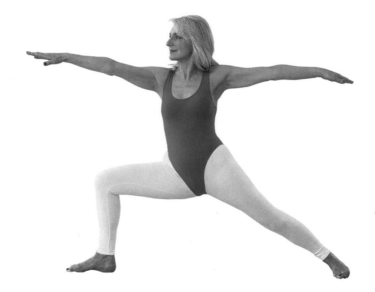

- Stand with your legs about 3½–4 ft apart and turn your right foot 90° to the right and have your left foot facing towards. Stretch your arms outwards and parallel to the floor.
- Inhale deeply and as you exhale bend your right leg aiming eventually to have your right thigh parallel to the floor and the left one straight.
- Ensure that the outer edge of your left foot stays on the floor and fix your gaze on the centre of your right hand.
- Hold your maximum stretch in this movement for a count of 5, lengthening the hold to a count of 10 as you become more adept at the movement.
- Inhale and return to an upright position.
- Exhale, relax and repeat to the other side.
- Repeat the entire sequence.

### *Extra Help*

*In the beginning stages, although this movement looks easy you may find it very difficult to keep your outer portion of your left leg on the floor. This is quite normal and again it will come with practice. Also, trying to have your thigh flat and your left leg straight can be a huge problem to start with but this pose slims and streamlines your thighs and calves and keeps them in great shape for life. I really recommend it.*

## STAGE 2

This movement has all the benefits of the previous posture but it also relieves tightness in the chest and neck and firms and tones the jaw and throat, and corrects posture.

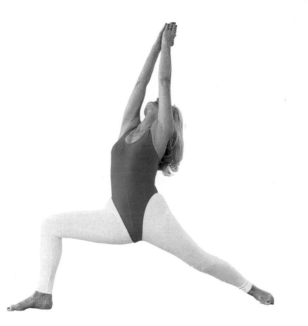

- Stand straight with your legs 3½–4 ft apart. Turn your right foot at 90° to the right and have your left foot facing forwards. Drop your head back and stretch your arms above your head, placing them together and cross your thumbs.
- Breathe in deeply and, as you exhale, bend your right leg again aiming your thigh flat and your back leg straight. Keep your gaze on your hands and breathe normally in your maximum position. Hold for a count of 5, increasing to 10 as you improve in the movement.
- Repeat on the other side and then repeat the entire sequence.

*Extra Help*
*Sometimes dropping your head back and looking at your hands is difficult so just do your best; it is a great tension reliever and an excellent aid to correcting poor posture.*

### TAKE 2 MINUTES: beauty tip

**Line-smoothing face mask** – This is brilliant, your lines and wrinkles just smooth away! If your face looks puffy or stressed before an important event, this mask will help. Cleanse your face thoroughly, then whisk 1 egg white with a few drops of lemon juice and apply it to the skin like a mask, being careful to avoid the eye area. Lie down and breathe slowly and calmly and leave the mask to harden (about 10 minutes). Remove with warm water then apply your moisturizer and make up as usual.

# DAY 3

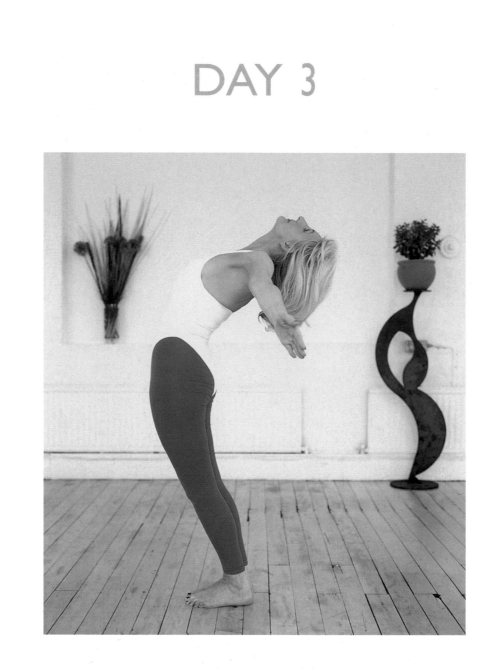

6 *Today is a new day. You will get out of it just what you put into it. If you have made mistakes, even serious mistakes, there is always another chance for you. And supposing you have tried and failed again and again. You may have a fresh start any moment you choose, for this anything we call 'failure' is not the falling down but the staying down.* 9

MARY PICKFORD

## TAKE 2 MINUTES: to focus on your goals

Remember to focus on your goals and your picture and visualize your beautiful lean toned shape – you are doing well and together we will get there.

Sit calmly and visualize a really great day ahead. Use today to practice and focus on feeling calm and peaceful inside. Whatever people say or do, be determined to stay calm.

*❝Nowhere can man find a quieter or more untroubled retreat than in his own soul.❞*

MARCUS AURELIUS

## TAKE 1 MINUTE: for today's menu

### Breakfast

½ grapefruit, 1 slice wholegrain toast
with a little butter,
1 boiled egg

### Lunch

4 oz cold poached salmon and large mixed salad
(use watercress, lettuce, cucumber,
chicory and a few pine nuts)
and 1 tbsp dressing (*see* recipe page 170)

1 bowl raspberries

### Dinner

Pork steak with red apples (*see* recipe page 166)
served with spinach and swede

# 1  Free the spirit

This movement gives you instant stress relief, literally making you feel free from all limitations. It is great if you have been sat at your desk for any length of time. It also helps correct your posture, releases shoulder tension and firms the throat and jaw line.

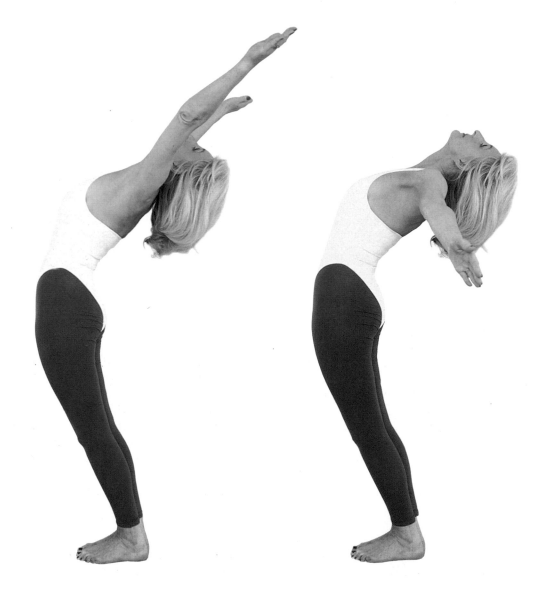

- Stand straight, shoulders back, feet together and correct your posture, hands in prayer.
- Inhale and lift your arms up straight in front of you until they are pointing to the ceiling.
- Drop your head gently backwards and

keeping it back, open your arms wide and making the widest circle possible lower your arms down to your sides while exhaling very slowly.
- Repeat three times.

# 2  Body roll

This simple tension-releasing movement does wonders for your waistline while relieving lower back tension.

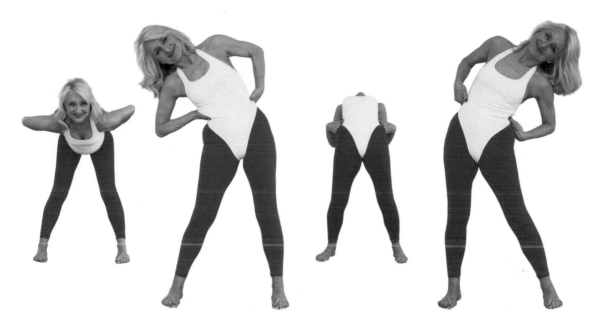

- Stand straight with your feet facing forwards and about 12 in apart.
- Place your hands at your waistline with your thumbs in front and fingers behind.
- Inhale deeply and, as you exhale, move slowly forwards keeping your head up.
- Breathing normally, slowly and carefully in continuous motion roll your body to the right, then carefully backwards, then to the left and slowly forwards. Do two circles to the right followed by two circles to the left.
- After completing the body roll, inhale deeply. Stand straight and stretch your arms straight up above your head. Place your hands together and straighten your spine. Hold the stretch for a count of 5, then exhale and slowly lower your arms and relax.

**Extra Help**
*The body roll is such a nice, easy exercise, it rarely presents any problems. Just remember to start with a small circle and expand it as your flexibility improves – always finish by stretching to realign the spine.*

# 3  Awkward posture

This important movement firms and tones your thighs while increasing the flexibility of your feet, knees and ankles.

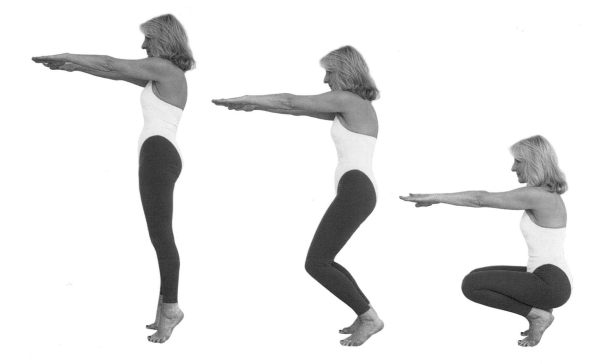

- Stand straight with your feet about 1 ft apart, your toes pointing forwards.
- Place your arms parallel to the floor.
- Inhale and gently come up on to your toes and, as you exhale, keeping your back straight, slowly lower your bottom to your heels. Please don't worry if only half way is possible to begin with. Move at your own pace without strain.
- Hold your maximum position in the movement for a count of 5. Then inhale and gradually return to an upright position keeping your back straight.
- Exhale, relax and repeat the movement twice.

### Extra Help
*It can be very disturbing suddenly to discover that your knees, feet and ankles have stiffened up. Again the 'use it or lose it' principle applies here. Cheer up – even if your joints are very stiff, a little practice a day does work wonders.*

# 4   Toe balance

This movement helps your sense of balance and concentration and strengthens the toes and arches of your feet.

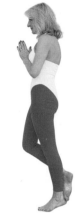

- Stand straight and place your hands in prayer.
- Place your right foot behind your left ankle. Breathe in and gently come up on to your toes. Exhale and hold the position, staring at a spot on the wall or floor to help you to balance for a count of 5, breathing normally.
- Lower your heel down to the floor, relax and repeat on the other side. Then repeat the entire sequence twice. Increase the hold to a count of 10 as you progress in the movement

### Extra Help

*I know this looks so simple and yet you can't do it. You wobble around or find it difficult to lift your heel from the floor. Again this is quite normal; stay calm and concentrate on that spot and gradually you will find your sense of balance and your feet strengthening. Yoga teaches us that the mind is like the sun's rays, normally they shine on all of us and give us warmth but concentrate them on one spot and they are powerful enough to cause fire. The mind likewise, when it concentrates on one thing at a time becomes extremely powerful, all the minor thoughts and worries of daily life start to vanish and your mind becomes clear and calm.*

## TAKE 2 MINUTES: beauty tip

**Dry skin brushing –** This is one of the best ways of shifting cellulite and improving lymphatic drainage. It also makes you look and feel better, your skin will look clearer and your eyes brighter. Do it before you bath or shower. It will take only about 2 minutes. Take a body brush or loofah and, starting at your feet, brush with long strokes in the direction of your heart. Do your legs, thighs, torso, front and back and then your arms, finger tips upwards, then with long downward strokes brush your neck and chest in the direction of your heart. Make sure you brush carefully, never redden your skin and never brush over cut or grazed skin.

After skin brushing, take a shower, finish with a cold rinse and massage yourself with your favourite body cream. You will feel great and tingle all over!

# DAY 4

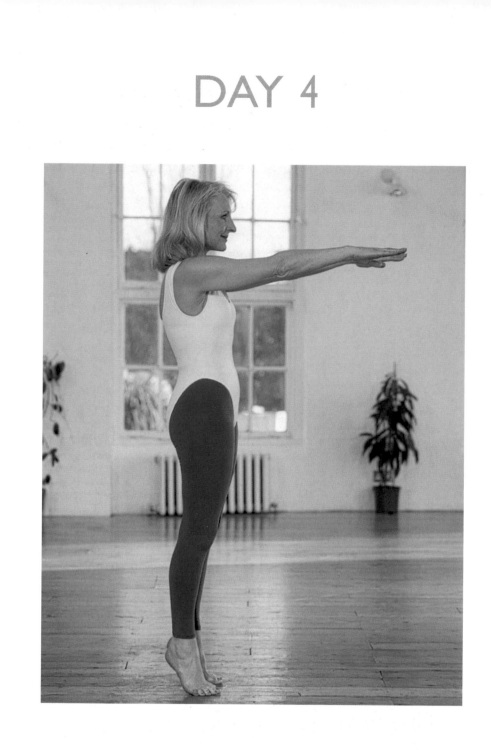

❝ *Make one person happy each day and in forty
years you will have made 14,600 human beings
happy for a little time at least.* ❞
CHARLES WILEY

## TAKE 2 MINUTES: to focus on your goals

Visualize your lovely slim beautiful body. Focus on your goals and keep them in your mind – make sure you are sticking to your plan and make at least one person happy today. Sit and visualize today's challenges turning out fine and see the way ahead going really well.

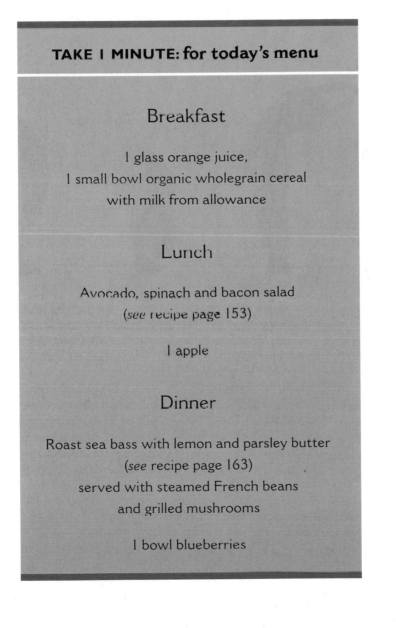

### TAKE 1 MINUTE: for today's menu

## Breakfast

1 glass orange juice,
1 small bowl organic wholegrain cereal
with milk from allowance

## Lunch

Avocado, spinach and bacon salad
(*see* recipe page 153)

1 apple

## Dinner

Roast sea bass with lemon and parsley butter
(*see* recipe page 163)
served with steamed French beans
and grilled mushrooms

1 bowl blueberries

DAY FOUR

# 1  Half-moon posture

I am so grateful to this position – it has helped me maintain my 24" waistline so that on my 60th birthday it was the same as it was on my 18th! It will do the same for you: it will whittle your waistline, remove your spare tyre and tone up your midriff both front and back and keep your spine tremendously flexible.

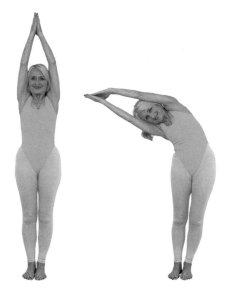

- Stand straight with your feet together. Inhale and lift your arms in the air placing your palms together and cross your thumbs. Stretch your arms upwards straightening them and place the insides of your upper arms on your ears.
- As you exhale, move slowly to the right pushing your hips a little to the left. Keep your body in line – don't move forwards or backwards. Hold for a count of 5, breathing normally, then slowly inhale and return to an upright position.
- Exhale as you move to the left, pushing your hips to the right. Hold for a count of 5, then inhale and return to an upright position.
- Exhale and bend forwards with your head up,

keeping your back flat and your legs straight, and relax in your maximum forwards bend without strain. Eventually aim to place your hands by your feet and your chin on your shins. Hold your maximum position for a count of 5 breathing normally.
- Inhale slowly, lift your head and arms and gently return to an upright position, stretching your arms up above your head.
- Now concentrate on your thumbs, gently bend backwards with a full lung. Exhale in your maximum backwards bend and hold for maximum movement for a count of 5.
- Inhale and return to an upright position. Exhale, relax and repeat.

### Extra Help
*Doesn't it look simple! Even standing straight with your head between your arms can be quite a challenge. Please just go at your own pace, if you can only move a little from side to side and for- wards and back to start with that is fine. You will still benefit and as you start to do the movement on a regular basis, your waist measurement will show you that it is working!*

# 2   Straight leg triangle

The triangle works the entire body toning the spinal nerves, firming and toning all the muscles around the abdomen, midriff, waistline, legs, arms and shoulders. It rids your spine of tension and gives it tremendous flexibility. This movement is excellent for the lower back and can help relieve lower backache. The backwards bend relieves tightness in the chest and tones the throat and jaw.

- Stand straight with your legs about 3½–4 ft apart.
- Turn your right foot 90° to the right, keep your left foot facing forwards, stretch your arms outwards at shoulder level, parallel to the floor: make sure that your legs stay straight throughout this movement.

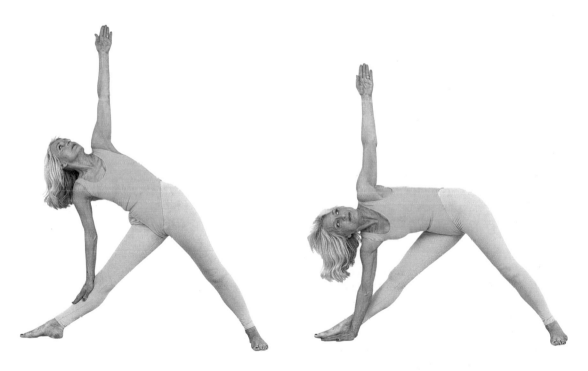

## STAGE 1

- Inhale and facing over your right leg, exhale, slowly lower your right hand to the floor aiming to place your right hand by your right foot with your little finger by your big toe. If this is not possible, don't bend your knee, simply hold your knee, calf or ankle. Now gently pull your left shoulder back, lift your left arm in the air keeping both arms in a straight line, and gently look at your left hand.
- Hold this movement for a count of 5, increasing to 10 as you progress in the posture.
- Inhale as you return to an upright position. Exhale and relax. Repeat to the left side.

## STAGE 2

- With your feet about 3½–4 ft apart and your arms parallel to the floor, inhale and change your arms over so that your left hand faces over your right foot.
- Exhale and keeping your legs straight aim to place your left thumb by your right big toe or again if this is not possible simply hold your knee, ankle or calf and lift your right arm in the air.

- Carefully rotate your trunk so that you are gazing at your right hand and aim to have both arms in line with each other.
- Hold your maximum position in this movement for a count of 5 increasing to 10 as you progress.
- Inhale and lift your left arm from the floor and carefully return to an upright position.
- Exhale, relax and repeat on the other side.
- Repeat the entire movement once.

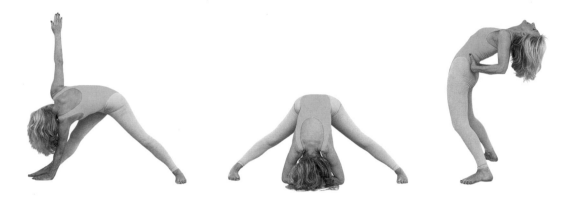

## STAGE 3

- With your legs 3–4 ft apart stand straight and ensure that your toes face forwards.
- Inhale and stretch both arms up in the air. Keeping your back flat and your legs straight, exhale and relax gently forwards into your maximum position.
- Just let go in this stretch and you will find that simply by relaxing in it you are able to move further into the posture. Eventually you will be able to fold your arms and place your elbows on the floor and rest your head on your arms. In the meantime, enjoy the movement and place your hands on your legs in your maximum stretch.
- Hold your best position for a count of 5,

increasing to 10 as you improve. Carefully draw your feet inwards until they are only 3 ft apart.
- Inhale and lifting your head first, slowly return to an upright position and stretch your arms up above your head, exhale and relax.
- Place your hands at your waistline with your fingers behind and thumbs in front.
- Now inhale deeply and gently bend backwards, exhale in your maximum position and hold your backwards bend for a count of 5, increasing gradually to 10 as you progress.
- Inhale and slowly return to an upright position. Exhale and relax.

### Extra Help

This movement frequently shows up your stiff areas. The most important point is to go carefully at your own pace and *relax* in your maximum movement. This way your stiffness will be eased gently and the movement will help your flexibility.

# 3 Tree balance

This movement does wonders for the joints in your legs; it literally oils your hips, knees, ankles and feet. It tones and firms all the muscles in your legs and is excellent for helping to prevent arthritis and rheumatism in your joints. It also helps your powers of concentration, balance and patience.

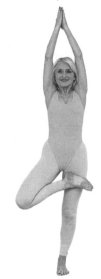

- Stand straight with your feet together and lift your right foot on to your left thigh (if this is difficult for you just place your foot in a comfortable position on your ankle, calf or thigh).
- Staring at a spot to enable you to balance, inhale and lift your arms straight up in the air, place your palms together and cross your thumbs.
- Hold this position for a count of 5, increasing to 10 as your strength improves.
- Exhale, lower your arms and leg, place your hands together and relax and repeat on the other side, then repeat the entire movement.

## Extra Help

Stiff hips, knees and ankles are the main problems here. Concentrate on your spot and even if you start by placing your foot on your ankle, that's fine. Daily practice will help relieve this stiffness and give you back your youthful flexibility.

---

### TAKE 2 MINUTES: beauty tip

**Nothing ruins your looks more than stress** – If you are really stressed and your life is in turmoil, sit quietly and breathe slowly and deeply, exhaling slowly after each breath. Now imagine that the sea is really rough, but you are lying on an unsinkable life raft. Inside you are calm and peaceful and can cope with anything, you are going to be fine. Keep this in your mind and relax, relax, relax.

# DAY 5

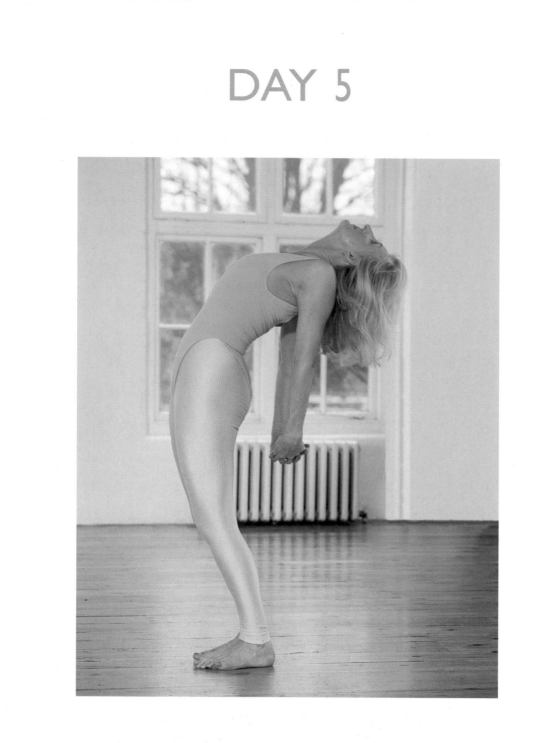

*We are all in the gutter but some of us are looking at the stars.*

OSCAR WILDE

## TAKE 2 MINUTES: to focus on your goals

Well done – it is Day 5. Keep focusing on your goals (or your stars) and your picture. You are doing really well to have got this far. Think about that beautiful new outfit you will be able to buy and just imagine how good you will feel in it. Visualize a great day ahead, see each meeting going well and everything working out for the best. Close your eyes and take each event one at a time and visualize a successful outcome.

## TAKE 1 MINUTE: for today's menu

### Breakfast

1 smoothie – blend 1 carton organic natural
yoghurt with 1 banana,
1 small carton raspberries and 1 tsp of honey

### Lunch

endive, walnut and blue cheese salad
(*see* recipe page 153)

2 figs

### Dinner

grilled fillets of lemon sole sprinkled with
fresh mixed herbs, mashed celeriac
(*see* recipe page 168), served with tomato,
basil and onion salad (*see* recipe page 154)

10 grapes

# 1   Salute to the sun

This is a very beautiful exercise routine in 12 parts. Traditionally, it should be done facing the sunrise. The sun was worshipped in ancient times and thought to be the giver of health and long life. A totally energizing routine, 'Salute to the Sun' stretches, tones and firms the muscles in the arms and legs, reduces abdominal flab, keeps the spine flexible, promotes healthy deep breathing and helps the circulation. This does wonders for the whole body, maintaining that youthful flexibility and energy and keeping it in excellent shape. Try to do the whole routine twice alternating which leg you take back first in position 4.

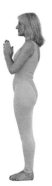
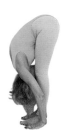
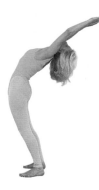

1   Stand straight, feet together, breathe in deeply and exhale slowly.

2   Raising your arms above your head, take a deep breath in and bend backwards. (Beginners may find it more comfortable to have their feet about 1 ft apart in this movement.)

3   Breathe out as you bend forwards, aiming your head to your knees and your hands by your feet. Aim to have the knees straight, but, if necessary, bend them in the beginning stages.

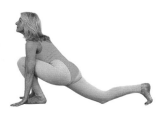
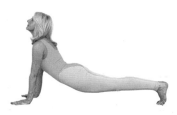
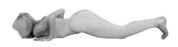

4   Breathe in as you stretch your right leg back from the body, keeping the left leg between the hands, and look upwards.

5   Breathe out and stretch your left leg back.

6   Lower the whole body on the floor. Knees first, then chest, then chin. Toes curled under.

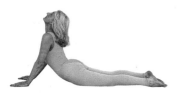

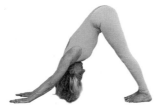

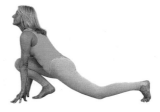

7  Lie completely flat. Breathe in and slowly come up to the Cobra position, lifting head, shoulders and upper body from the floor and dropping your head back (*see* page 64).

8  Exhale and lift your bottom up in the air as you drop your head and shoulders, keeping your hands flat on the floor.

9  Breathe in, and bring your right foot in between your hands.

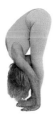

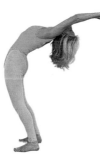

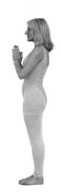

10  Breathe out, bring your left foot in and look up. Then lift your bottom in the air and aim the head to the knees.

11  Breathe in and slowly come up into an upright position raising your arms and bending backwards.

12  Exhale, drop your arms and place them in prayer and relax.

## TAKE 2 MINUTES: beauty tip

**Walk tall with correct posture** – This makes such a difference to the way you look and feel. Good posture can make you look 10 years younger. Stand in front of a long mirror, lift your chin and stand straight with your feet together. Now, take a piece of hair on top of your head and pull it upwards. Walk forwards 6 paces and see how much straighter you feel. Alternatively, adopt the old-fashioned system of walking with 2 books balanced on the top of your head. Either way it will correct your posture and prevent you from stooping.

# DAY 6

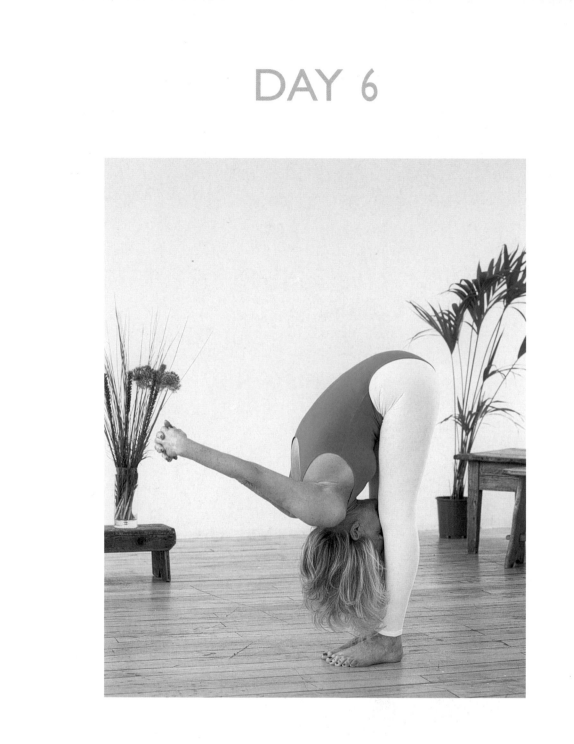

*Wake up with a smile and go after life.
Live it, enjoy it, taste it, smell it, feel it.*

JOE KNAPP

## TAKE 2 MINUTES: to focus on your goals

Well, we are nearly at the end of Week 1 so keep on focusing on your goals and tomorrow we will measure Week 1 results. Today, think about your summer holiday and see yourself looking fabulous in a lovely new bikini! Visualize your lovely day ahead. Try to do something new today, maybe pick up some brochures and think about your next holiday. Treat yourself to a few lovely flowers. Just make it a great day.

## TAKE 1 MINUTE: for today's menu

### Breakfast

½ grapefruit, 1 slice of toast topped
with 4 grilled tomatoes

### Lunch

prawn salad (*see* recipe page 154)

½ banana

### Dinner

4 oz roast turkey breast, 1tsp cranberry sauce,
4 roast parsnip chunks, 2 tbsp Brussels sprouts,
1 tbsp gravy

2 kiwi fruit

# TAKE 25 MINUTES: for today's exercises

Today, take the time to go through *all* the movements you have learned so far. This will take you about 25 minutes.

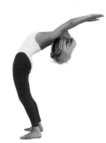

- Upwards stretch forwards and backwards bend

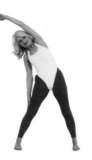

- Sideways stretch

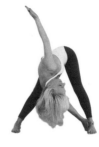

- Rishi's posture

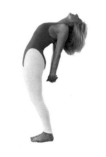

- Chest expansion

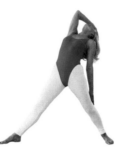

- Siamese posture

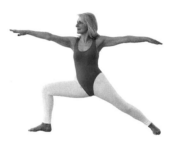

- Warrior posture

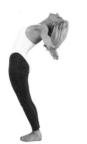

- Free the spirit

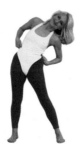

- Body roll

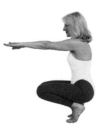

- Awkward posture

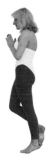

• Toe balance

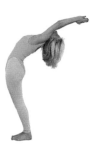

• Half-moon posture

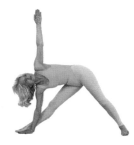

• Straight leg triangle

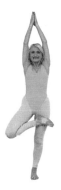

• Tree balance

• Salute to the Sun

## TAKE 2 MINUTES: beauty tip

**To remove eye bags** – Put a thin layer of haemorrhoid cream on them and leave for 10–15 minutes. Clean off with eye make-up remover. It works like magic.

*Caution:* Please note this is an emergency measure only. Do not use more than once every 2 weeks!

# DAY 7

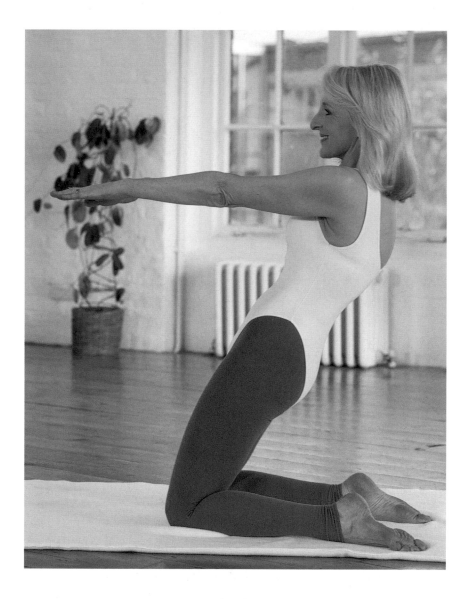

❛ *You should nurse your dreams and protect them through bad times and tough times to the sunshine and light which always come* ❜

WOODROW WILSON

## TAKE 2 MINUTES: to focus on your goals

Well done! You have now made it through Week 1. Now it's time to weigh and measure your-self and enter these into your notebook. You should have lost 2–3 lbs this week, so make sure your fridge is stocked with wonderful fresh and healthy foods for Week 2.

## TAKE 1 MINUTE: for today's menu

### Breakfast

1 small carton strawberries, 1 pot natural yoghurt

### Lunch

4 oz or 2 slices roast beef, 1 tsp horseradish sauce, steamed carrots and French beans, 1 tbsp gravy

½ cantaloupe melon

### Dinner

4 oz or 3 slices cold turkey, 1 tbsp celeriac in mustard mayonnaise, green salad

1 peach

## TAKE 25 MINUTES: for today's exercises

No exercises today, so get out in the fresh air and have a wonderful stroll around a park.

## TAKE 2 MINUTES: beauty tip

**To refresh your face** – When your skin feels tired, take a face flannel, soak it in warm water, ring it out and place it over the whole of your face. Leave it on for ½ minute, remove and repeat. Finally, repeat with cold water. Cleanse, moisturize and reapply your make up.

# DAY 8

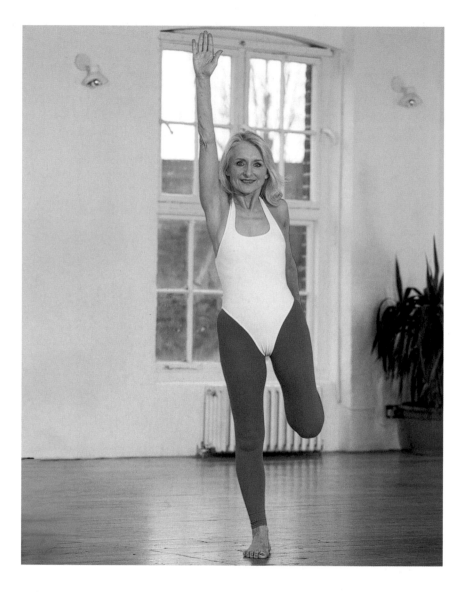

6 *Man is fond of counting his troubles, but he does not count his joys. If he counted them up as he ought to, he would see that every lot has enough happiness provided for it.* 9

FYODOR DOSTOYEVSKY

# TAKE 2 MINUTES: to focus on your goals

Spend a moment focusing on your goals – visualize your perfect shape, think of the lovely new clothes you will be able to wear and visualize yourself wearing them. Give thanks for your health, friends, family and your many blessings. In your notebook start a list of your blessings: begin with 5.

> *The best way for a person to have happy thoughts is to count his blessings not his cash.*
>
> ANON

---

## TAKE 1 MINUTE: for today's menu

### Breakfast

4 oz glass cranberry juice, 1 poached egg on
1 slice wholegrain toast

### Lunch

Greek salad (*see* recipe page 154)

1 peach

### Dinner

2 grilled herrings and lemon slices, served with
steamed broccoli and carrots

1 bowl of raspberries

**Caution: Do not attempt these movements if you're pregnant**

# 1  Abdominal lift

The abdominals drop as we get older and this movement is invaluable for keeping the abdomen firm, toned, uplifted and youthful. It takes 30 seconds a day and is brilliant! This movement must be done on an empty stomach. The ideal time to do it is before breakfast.

10 MINUTES IN THE MORNING

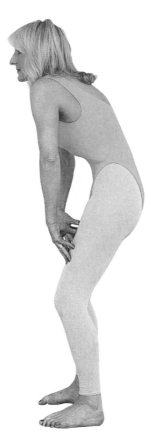

- Stand straight with your legs about 1 ft apart and place your hands on your upper thighs.
- Inhale deeply then exhale fully and, keeping the air out of your lungs, pull your abdominals in and up.

- Hold for a count of 10. Release the abdominals, inhale and relax.
- Repeat the movement twice.

### Extra Help
*Please don't worry if you don't appear to get much movement in the beginning stages, just persevere – the result of a slimmer, firmer and flatter stomach is well worth it!*

# 2   Tummy and thigh toner

This powerful movement really tones and firms your tummy. It gives your thighs that beautiful firm, toned, slim yoga shape. This deceptively simple movement is like dynamite!

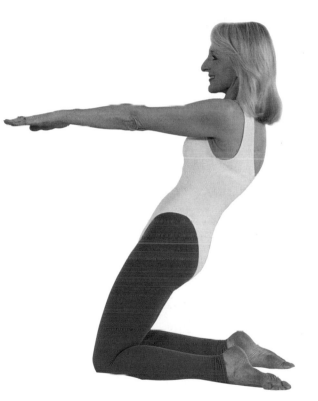

DAY EIGHT

- Kneel with your knees about 1 ft apart.
- Lift your bottom from your heels and place your arms parallel to the floor making sure that your thighs are straight and perpendicular to the floor.
- Inhale and as you exhale just lean back a

small way, at first increasing the stretch as you progress in the movement – don't allow your bottom to sag. Hold the position for a count of 5, breathing normally, then inhale and return to an upright position and repeat twice.

# 3   Pose of a boat

This is a fantastic firmer for both tummies and thighs and also greatly strengthens the lower back.

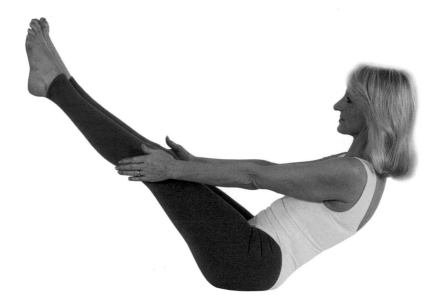

## STAGE 1

- Sit straight with both legs straight out in front of you, making sure that you are sitting on a nice thick mat or blanket.
- Place your arms parallel to the floor.
- Inhale and as you exhale gently lift your legs from the floor and balance on your bottom. Hold just for a count of 1 to begin with, gradually increasing the hold to 10 as you progress in the movement, then gently lower your legs to the floor, relax and repeat twice. This can be hard work but move carefully and build it up gently, and remember never strain in the posture.
- Following the movement, lie on your back, draw your knees to your chest and gently rock your back from side to side to relieve any tension in your lower back.

40

## STAGE 2

Again it is a powerful toner for your abdomen, thighs and lower back. Please don't ever attempt this movement until you can hold 'Pose of a boat – stage 1' for at least a count of 5.

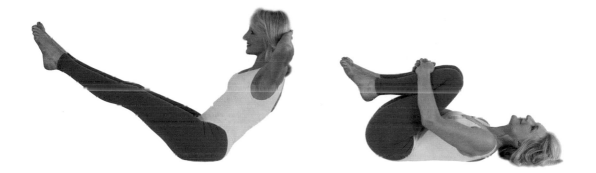

- Sitting on your mat with both legs stretched out in front of you, place your hands interlocked behind your head.
- Take a deep breath and, as you exhale, lift both your legs gently from the floor. Hold for a count of one to start with and then again increase gradually as you practice until you are holding for a count of 10. This is very powerful – don't strain! Gently lower your legs to the floor, then relax and repeat twice.
- Following the movement, lie down and gently draw your knees to your chest and rock from side to side.

---

### TAKE 2 MINUTES: beauty tip

**To lift and firm your bottom** – And also tone and strengthen your pelvic floor muscles. Stand straight with your feet about 1 ft apart and simply squeeze tight your pelvic floor muscles as though you are preventing yourself from passing urine. At the same time squeeze tight your buttock muscles, hold for 5 then release. Do 10 a day to start with, increasing to 30 with practice. This is easy to fit into your life, do a few at the photocopier or while waiting in a queue. If you do it slowly, no one will see but you will be delighted with the results.

# DAY 9

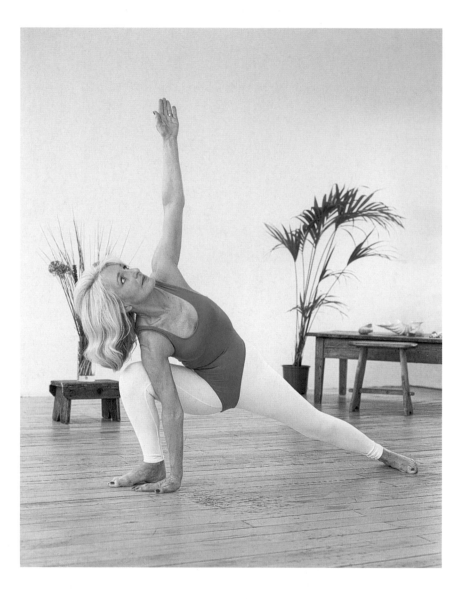

❝ *All our dreams can come true if we have the courage to pursue them.* ❞
WALT DISNEY

## TAKE 2 MINUTES: to focus on your goals

Spend a minute focusing on your goals, visualize your new slim body. You are doing really well to have got this far. Visualize a lovely day ahead. Take time to see if you can add any more changes to make your life better. Perhaps you could listen to beautiful music as you do the dishes or light scented candles and have some fresh flowers on your dinner table. Remember, it is the tiny changes that can make your life more beautiful. Add 2 more things to your blessings list.

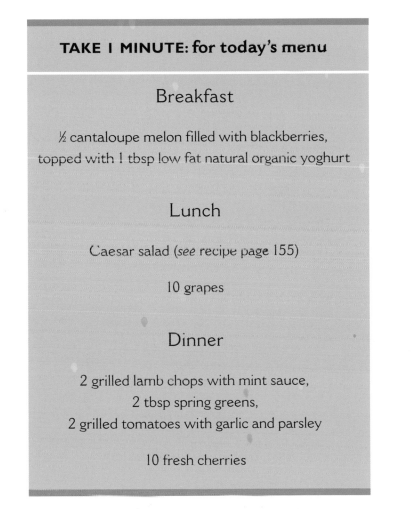

### TAKE 1 MINUTE: for today's menu

## Breakfast

½ cantaloupe melon filled with blackberries, topped with 1 tbsp low fat natural organic yoghurt

## Lunch

Caesar salad (*see* recipe page 155)

10 grapes

## Dinner

2 grilled lamb chops with mint sauce,
2 tbsp spring greens,
2 grilled tomatoes with garlic and parsley

10 fresh cherries

# 1   Pose of a mountain

This is excellent for releasing neck and shoulder tension, it firms and tones the upper arms and is invaluable for correcting posture.

## STAGE 1

- Kneel down with your bottom on your heels (if this is difficult, place a cushion between your bottom and heels).
- Interlock your hands in front of you; now turn them inside out so that you are looking at the backs of your hands.
- Inhale and lift your arms up above your head ensuring that the 'inside' of your arms are in line with your ears, your back is straight and your hands are directly above your head.
- Hold this position for a count of 5, breathing normally, then exhale, lower your arms and relax. Repeat 3 times.

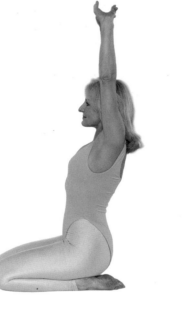 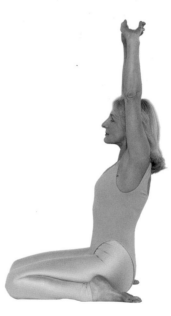

## STAGE 2

When, and only when, you can sit on your heels with ease then you may try this more advanced stage of the movement. This is so good for keeping your knees and hips flexible and is excellent for correcting poor posture and straightening your back.

- In a high kneeling position, open your knees hip width apart. Place your hands on your heels and carefully and without strain, aim to lower your bottom to the floor between your heels.
- When this kneeling position is possible, interlock your hands in front of you and lift your arms in the air as in the previous position.
- Hold for a count of 5, breathing normally, then undo your arms, relax and repeat three times.

# 2   Pose of a cow

This movement, although humbling at first as it can show how stiff and imbalanced your shoulders have become, is fantastic. This movement is invaluable for rebalancing the shoulders, releasing shoulder tension, correcting posture and firming and toning your upper arms. Stage 2 is excellent for aiding the flexibility and tone of your hips, knees and ankles.

## STAGE 1

- Sit on your heels (use a cushion if this is not yet comfortable for you).
- Inhale deeply and lift your left arm in the air and drop it back over your left shoulder.
- Take your right arm up and behind your back and try to join both arms together. Hold your maximum position in this movement for a count of 5. (Don't worry if your hands are still a long way apart – with practice you will improve). Unclasp your hands, relax and repeat on the other side. Do notice if you find

it easier on one side and difficult on the other; these imbalances can be caused by many things including heavy shoulder bags that can weigh down one shoulder or constant use of the right arm as opposed to the left one. The imbalances are important and this movement is invaluable as it will rebalance your shoulders.

It is also an excellent movement for the lungs as it helps open them fully.

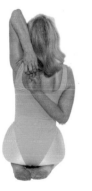 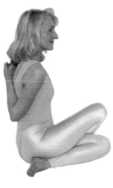 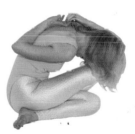

## STAGE 2

- Once you can sit with ease in a kneeling position with your bottom on your heels then you may try the full cow posture.
- In a high kneeling position, place your hands on the floor.
- Cross your right leg over your left and ensure that your heels are hip width apart. Inhale then as you exhale and keeping your weight on your hands, carefully lower your bottom between your heels aiming to sit comfortably in this position. Place your hands on your upper knee and relax. If you can't yet manage this position don't worry, just repeat Stage 1.

- Sitting in this position, inhale and lift your right arm in the air, take your left arm back behind your back and try to clasp them together. Then exhale and bend forwards and aim your head to touch your upper knee. Hold this position breathing normally for a count of 8, then inhale and return to an upright position. Exhale, relax and repeat to the other side.

Again, please note that the leg movement may be much easier one side than the other.

**45**

# 3  Sideways body raise

This is an excellent movement for firming and toning the upper arms, stretching out tension in the wrist and hands and strengthening the arms, so helping to prevent osteoporosis. When we fall, it is an automatic response to extend a hand or arm to break the fall. If the arms are weak this can easily lead to a sprain or fracture.

**Note:** if you have recently had an arm injury, follow the directions below but *do not lift your body from the floor*. Just put a little weight on your arms and wait until you have regained your strength before moving on to the full movement.

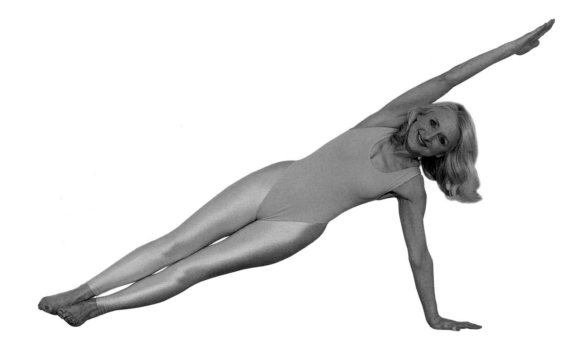

- Sit with both hands to the right side of your body and make sure that both your hands and feet are on a firm non-slip surface. Bend your knees.
- Inhale deeply and, as you exhale, lift your body from the floor and support it on both hands and feet.
- Now adjust your body so that your right shoulder is directly above your right wrist and your arm is straight.
- Lift your bottom and adjust your feet so that the left foot is placed on top of the right one and the body is in a straight line.

- When, and only when, you feel strong enough, lift your left arm from the floor and stretch it in a straight line with the inside of the arm alongside your left ear. Concentrate on a spot on the floor to help your balance and hold the movement for a count of 5, breathing normally.
- Gently lower your bottom to the floor and relax, repeat on the other side.
- Do the movement just once to begin with, but when you feel strong enough then perform the movement twice on each side.

# 4   Pose of a plane

A beautiful movement to tone and firm and strengthen the arms, wrists and hands and release lower back tension.

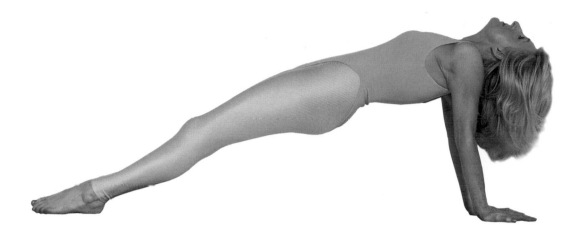

- Sit straight with your hands comfortably on the floor behind you with your fingertips facing backwards and your legs straight out on the floor in front of you. Ensure that both your hands and feet are on a non-slip surface.
- Inhale deeply and gently lift your body from the floor supporting your weight on your hands and your feet.
- Ensure that your body is in a straight line and

that your toes are on the floor. Allow your head to drop back and hold your maximum position breathing normally for a count of 5, increasing to 10 with practice.
- Slowly lower your body to the floor, relax and repeat once.
- Now lie down and draw your knees to your chest, interlock your hands around them and rock gently from left to right to relax your lower back.

---

### TAKE 2 MINUTES: beauty tip

**To firm a double chin –** Sit with your back straight and grin from ear to ear. Whilst grinning, gently drop your head back and, still grinning, slowly open and close your mouth three times. Repeat twice. Do it daily and see the difference.

# DAY 10

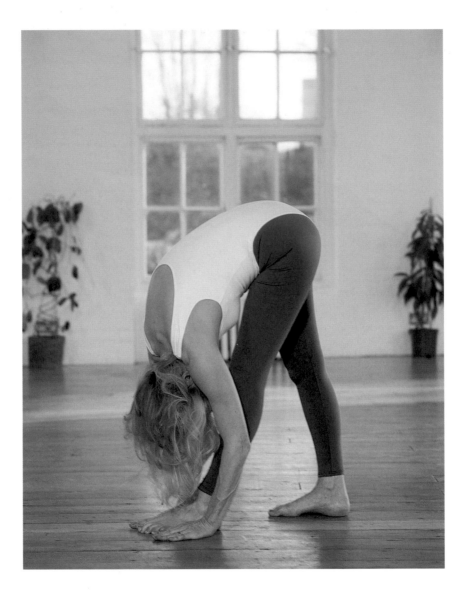

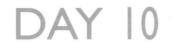 *Be glad of life because it gives you the chance to love and to work and to play and to look up at the stars.*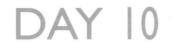

HENRY VAN DYKE

## TAKE 2 MINUTES: to focus on your goals

Never skip this vital step as the reason most people fail on any diet or indeed at any-thing is because it gradually goes out of their mind. You must daily visualize your dream and keep it exciting and alive but make sure you daily give thanks and be grateful for your blessings. Sit and visualize a beautiful, peaceful and stress-free day ahead.

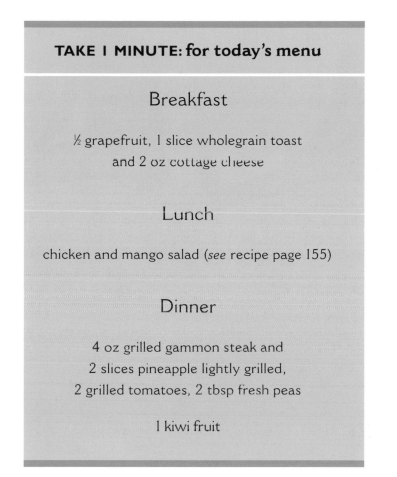

## TAKE 1 MINUTE: for today's menu

### Breakfast

½ grapefruit, 1 slice wholegrain toast
and 2 oz cottage cheese

### Lunch

chicken and mango salad (*see* recipe page 155)

### Dinner

4 oz grilled gammon steak and
2 slices pineapple lightly grilled,
2 grilled tomatoes, 2 tbsp fresh peas

1 kiwi fruit

# 1 Alternate leg pull

One of yoga's all-time greats! This movement ensures the flexibility of your feet, ankles, hips and thighs. It stretches and tones your hamstrings and calf muscles, rebalances your lower back and massages your lower abdominal organs.

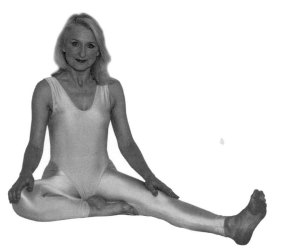

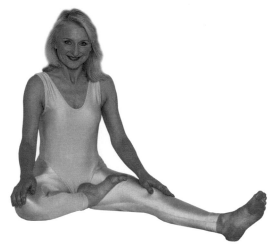

- Sit straight with both legs straight out in front of you.
- Carefully lift your right foot on to your left thigh
- Place your right hand onto your right knee
- Very gently and carefully bounce your knee towards the floor about 6 times. This movement will help you loosen your hip, knee and ankle.

- If your foot is comfortable on your thigh and your right knee is on the floor, then leave it there. If it isn't comfortable, place your right foot in the space between your legs with your heel in your groin.
- Inhale and lift both your arms in the air.

> *No-one succeeds without effort ... those who succeed owe their success to their perseverance.*
>
> RAMANA MAHARSHI

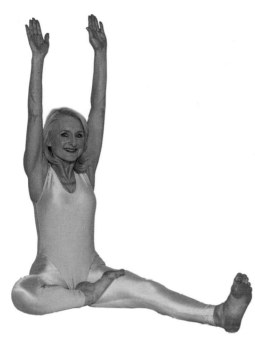

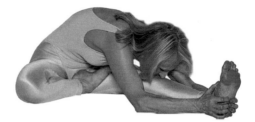

- Exhale and with your head up and back flat, bend forwards into your maximum position without strain. (Your eventual aim is to clasp your left foot and place your chin on your shin but, as always, your maximum position in the movement is fine.)
- Hold your maximum stretch for a count of 5, increasing to 10 as you progress in this position. Then inhale and slowly lift your head and arms and return to an upright position.

Exhale, relax and repeat the movement.
- Repeat on the other side this time bringing your left foot on to the right thigh and notice any imbalances in your body. Is one side easier than the other? Is one hip stiffer than the other? It is very important to notice these imbalances and carefully correct them or they can lead to problems in later life.

### Extra Help
*This movement can be a real eye-opener. Frequently your joints are stiffer than you think and one side of your body is very much easier than the other. These imbalances may be caused by a number of things from poor posture to imbalanced sports such as tennis or golf, which use one side of the body more than the other. However imbalanced or stiff you are, yoga can help put matters right. Practice daily and see the difference.*

# 2 Thigh stretch

This movement helps to keep the flexibility of the hip joints and tones and firms the inner thighs.

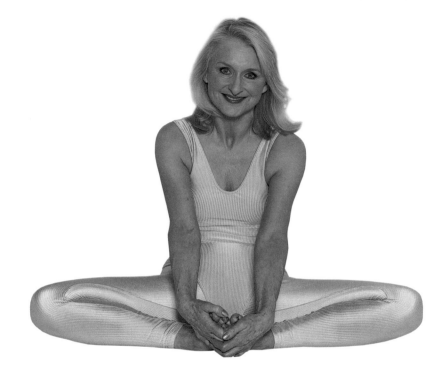

- Sit up straight and bring both your feet into the space between your legs. Place the soles of your feet together and interlock your hands around your toes.
- Take a deep breath in and, as you exhale, gently draw your knees towards the floor.

Hold your maximum stretch without straining and breathing normally for a count of 5, increasing to 10 as you progress in the movement.
- Inhale as you return your knees to an upright position. Exhale, relax and repeat three times.

### Extra Help
*This movement is so good for the health of the pelvic floor and flexibility of the hips, I can't recommend it too highly. Please don't worry if at first your knees are nowhere near the floor; just practice and see the difference.*

# 3   Pose of a star

A wonderful movement for releasing lower back tension, increasing the flexibility of your hips and promoting the health of the pelvic floor region. It is also excellent for toning and firming the inner thighs.

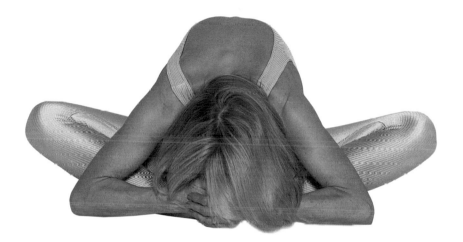

- Sit straight with both hands around soles of your feet and draw your feet towards your groin.
- Inhale deeply and as you exhale gently draw your knees towards the floor and then bend forwards into your maximum position without strain, eventually aiming your head to your toes.

- Breathing normally, hold your maximum position in this movement for a count of 5, increasing to 10 as you progress in it.
- Inhale, slowly return to an upright position, exhale, relax and repeat twice.

### Extra Help
*It is normal not to move far in this movement in the beginning stages, the hips are stiff and bending forwards can be quite difficult. Please remember, though, that you benefit at every stage in every yoga posture and with practice you will reach your goal. It feels so good when you do.*

# 4 The Lotus positions

I have to say it, this pose is not often comfortable to start with, but once your joints are sufficiently flexible for you to do it with ease, it honestly is very relaxing! It is recommended for breathing exercises and meditation, since the spine is erect and the legs entwined so that fidgeting is impossible and concentration is helped. It maintains incredible flexibility of the hips, knees and ankles.

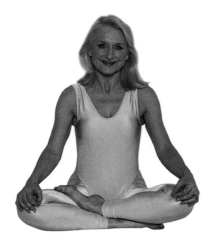

## The Half-Lotus Position

- Sit straight with both legs straight out in front of you and bring your right heel against your groin.
- Inhale and then gently try to lift your left foot onto your right thigh for the half-lotus position. (If you can't please don't worry, your flexibility will return and all yoga breathing exercises which advise a lotus position can easily be done in a crossed-legged position).
- Stay in this position for a count of 10, breathing slowly and deeply, then gently unwind your legs, stretch them out and try the movement with your right foot on your left thigh. Please note that in the beginning stages, one side is often easier than the other.

## The Full-Lotus Position

Once you can manage the half-lotus position, then it is time to try the full lotus.

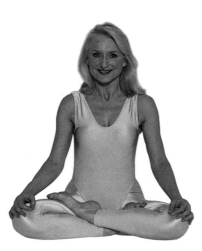

- Sit straight with both legs straight out in front of you and carefully aim to lift your right foot onto your left thigh, then gently and carefully lift your left foot onto your right thigh. (You may need to make several attempts at this before your joints are sufficiently flexible to achieve it, again just persevere without ever straining.) Once you are able to do the position, then stay in it for a count of 10, breathing calmly, slowly and deeply and then gently come out of it and repeat it, this time placing your left foot on to your right thigh to begin with and then your right foot onto the left thigh. Again, you will often find this position much easier with the legs one way rather than the other. It is, however, very important that you alternate your legs in this posture to ensure even and correct development of your flexibility.

**54**

## Lotus position with Twist

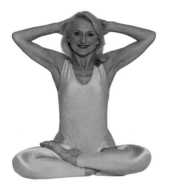

This is great for toning your midriff and waistline. It also removes tension from the lower back and increases spinal flexibility.

- Sit in either a cross-legged, half-lotus or full-lotus position.

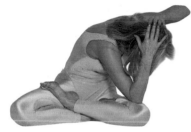

- Interlock your hands behind your head. Take a deep breath in and, as you exhale, gently take your right elbow to your left knee. Lifting the left elbow, aim to look behind you and hold this position breathing normally for a count of 5, then gently return to an upright position.

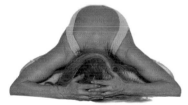

- Repeat on the other side then take a very deep breath and as you exhale, gently bend forwards aiming your head to the floor. Relax in this position for a count of 5, breathing normally. Inhale and return to an upright position, exhale, relax and repeat the entire sequence twice.

---

### TAKE 2 MINUTES: beauty tip

**To firm and tone your upper arms –** This is brilliant, and it also firms and tones your calves. Do it in the kitchen while waiting for the kettle to boil.

- Stand straight with feet about 1 ft apart (bare feet is best) about 2 ft away from your kitchen worktop.
- Place your hands on the worktop, fingers on top, thumbs underneath about 1 ft apart.

- Keeping your heels on the floor and your back straight, bend your elbows and lower your body towards the worktop.
- Straighten your arms as you gently return to your starting position. Do 5 times to begin with and build up slowly to 10, and then eventually to 25.

# DAY 11

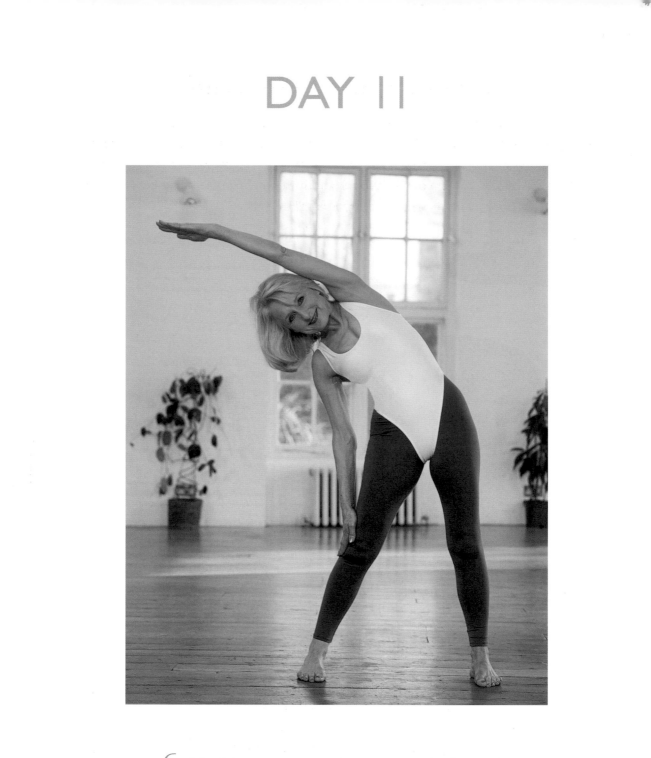

6 *Nothing can stop the man with the right mental attitude from achieving his goal, nothing on earth can help the man with the wrong mental attitude.* 9

W.W. ZIEGE

# TAKE 2 MINUTES: to focus on your goals

Get your notebook out and visualize your beautiful body goal. You are doing well to get this far so keep it up. Concentrate today on making a difficult relationship easier; visualize the person in question becoming calmer and easier to get on with. Try to compliment him or her on some aspect of their clothing or work or ask about their interests. Talk to this person as though you both had a great relationship and see the difference.

## TAKE 1 MINUTE: for today's menu

### Breakfast

½ cantaloupe melon filled with raspberries,
topped with 1 tbsp natural organic yoghurt

### Lunch

Make a sandwich, using 2 slices wholegrain bread
spread with a little butter, filled with 1 oz brie
thinly sliced, 1 sliced tomato, shredded lettuce,
few mixed salad sprouts

fresh blackberries

### Dinner

4 oz grilled chicken, 4 grilled mushrooms
with garlic and herbs, 2 grilled tomatoes,
carrot and apple salad (*see* recipe page 156)

1 fresh fig

Today's movements are great for your spine.

# 1 Back stretch

This is a yoga essential. It is perfect for stretching and realigning the spine, and for toning the back and the thighs. The back stretch releases tension in the lower back, stretches the hamstrings and tones the back of the thighs. It tones the abdominal area and rejuvenates the entire spine, massages the heart and is very relaxing.

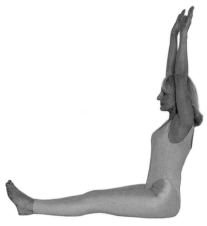

- Sit very straight with both legs straight out in front of you.

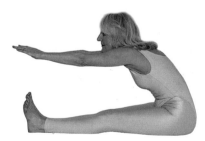

- Take a deep breath in and lift both your arms straight up in the air. Exhale as you gradually bend forwards with your head up and back flat, eventually aiming your chin to your knees. (When you first start this movement, you often find that your chin and knees are a long way apart. Please don't be discouraged, just keep practising and you will be amazed at how quickly you progress in the movement.)

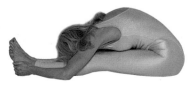

- Stay in your maximum position breathing normally for a count of 5.
- Inhale and slowly lift your head and arms and return to an upright position. Exhale and relax and repeat twice.

# 2   Simple twist

This gives great strength and flexibility to your spine while toning and firming your midriff, waistline and hips. The movement massages your internal organs stimulating the circulation to the kidneys, liver and spleen.

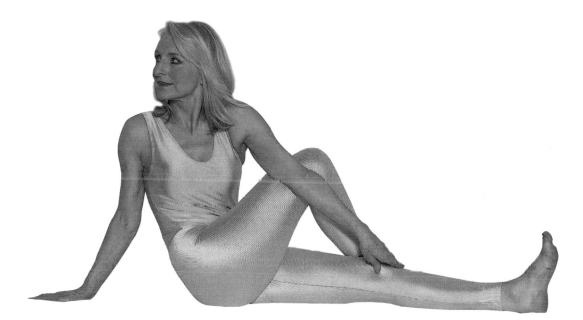

- Sit straight with both legs straight out in front of you.
- Lift your right leg over your left and place it on the floor on the outside of your left thigh.
- Inhale and place your right hand on the floor behind your back, then take your left arm on the outside of your right knee and place it on your left knee.

- Exhale slowly and, with perfect posture, rotate your torso to the right and turn your head over your right shoulder.
- Hold your maximum stretch in this position for a count of 5, increasing to 10 as you progress in the movement.
- Slowly return your head to the front and repeat. Perform the movement twice on the other side.

### Extra Help
*Sometimes it is not possible to take the right hand to the right knee at the beginning, so just let it rest in your maximum position. If twisting is difficult, don't push or strain, just do your best and with practice you will get there. You will really start to experience the benefits of the twist when you go to park your car!*

# 3  Wide-angled leg stretch

This does wonders for your shape, it really whittles your waist and tones up your midriff and inner thighs and is good for your back, especially the lumbar region. It is a boon to women as it can give tremendous help with menstrual problems.

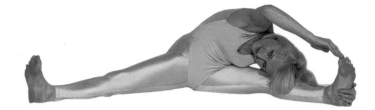

- Sit straight with your legs comfortably wide apart. Inhale and slide your left hand down your left leg towards your left heel, as you exhale bring your right arm alongside your right ear with your right hand eventually to your left foot. (This is the aim – remember just to go as far as you can without strain.) Relax in your maximum position for a count of 5.
- Inhale and slowly return to an upright position (exhale, relax and repeat on the other side).

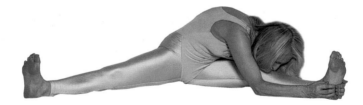

- Now sit with both arms parallel to your left leg, inhale and as you inhale bend forwards with your head up and a straight back and as you exhale gently try to clasp your left foot and move as far as you can eventually aiming your chin to your shin. Relax in your maximum stretch and hold it for a count of 5, then inhale, return to an upright position, exhale, relax and repeat on the other side.

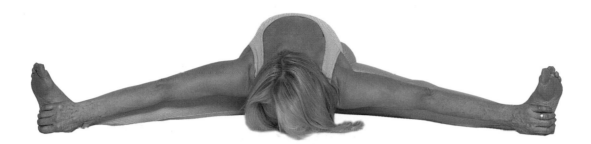

- Finally, sit straight with your legs comfortably wide apart, your arms parallel to your legs, inhale and as you exhale carefully stretch forwards keeping your head up and your back straight. Your eventual aim is to have your chin on the floor – this could take many months of practice but meanwhile you'll benefit tremendously in your maximum position. Relax and hold for a count of 5, increasing to 10 as you progress.

- Inhale and return to an upright position. Exhale, relax and repeat twice.

## Extra Help

*We have all been there! This position looks impossible – your chin is 3 ft from the floor and your legs won't even open wide. Please persevere, we all start like this and daily practice and patience are all you need to achieve the maximum stretch – and when you get there it feels great!*

## TAKE 2 MINUTES: beauty tip

### Get active!

1   At the supermarket, park your car furthest away from the entrance.
2   If your office is on the top floor, walk up 2 floors and then take the lift.
3   Get up to change the TV channel instead of using the remote control.
4   Always walk to the post box (provided it is not too far away!).
5   Run up and down stairs at home.

It's easy, just do it. It will help you lose weight, have more energy and make you feel like a much more energetic person.

# DAY 12

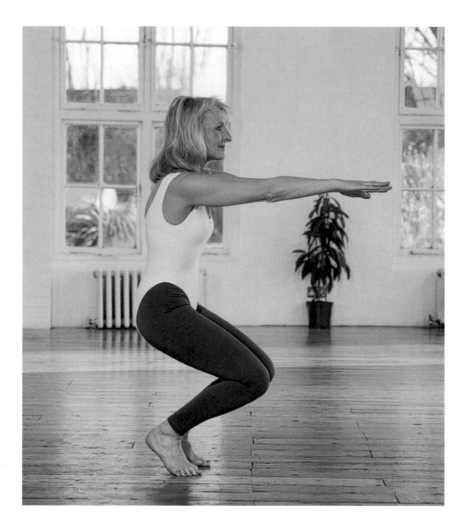

❝ *You can vitally influence your life from within by auto-suggestion. The first thing each morning, and the last thing each night. Suggest to yourself specific ideas that you wish to embody in your character and personality. Address such suggestions to yourself silently or aloud until they are deeply impressed upon your mind.* ❞

GRENVILLE KLEISER

## TAKE 2 MINUTES: to focus on your goals

Look at your goals and reassess them – we are moving in the right direction and it is good to check to see if the image you wrote down on Day 1 needs amending in any way. Maybe that now you are feeling better you could add another attribute that you would like to have or to change, to make it an even more dynamic and positive statement.

Now give thanks for your health, happiness and progress and add 3 more blessings to your list.

## TAKE 1 MINUTE: for today's menu

### Breakfast

1 small bowl organic muesli
with milk from allowance,
1 glass apple juice

### Lunch

mozzarella, tomato and basil salad
(*see* recipe page 156)

2 slices pineapple

### Dinner

4 oz roast breast of duck, 3 slices of orange,
2 tbsp mangetout, 2 tbsp carrot puree

1 fresh fig

# 1  Pose of a cobra

**Caution:** Do not do this movement during pregnancy.

This is so relaxing and ideal for before bedtime. It tones and strengthens your upper arms, wrists and hands; gives the spine tremendous flexibility and helps correct poor posture. It is excellent for helping to relieve menstrual cramps and backache. It tones the liver, spleen and kidneys, and stimulates the thyroid gland in the neck.

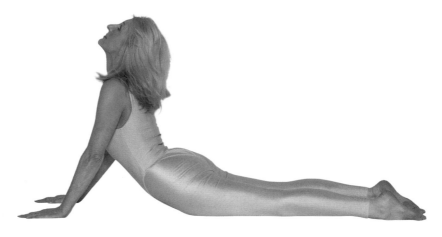

- Lie on your mat face down with your feet together and place your forehead on the floor. Your hands should be 3 in from your body with your fingers facing forwards and in line with your shoulders.
- Inhale deeply and, as you exhale, lift your head and place your chin on the floor.
- Inhale again and keeping your lower abdominals on the floor, lift your head and upper body slowly from the floor into your maximum stretch without strain. Drop your head back and exhale in your maximum position. Again, please don't worry if only a little movement is possible in the beginning stages.

- Hold your maximum position for a count of 5, breathing normally, increasing the hold to a count of 10 as your strength increases.
- Slowly lower yourself to the floor, place your forehead on the floor then turn your head on one side and relax. Repeat twice.
- Finish by inhaling and lifting your bottom in the air, exhale and stretch back onto to your heels keeping your arms at full stretch and relax in this position called 'pose of a swan' for a count of 5. Inhale and return to a kneeling position, stretch your arms up in the air crossing your hands, hold for 5, then lower them, exhale and relax.

### Extra Help
*This beautiful backwards curve of the body can be very difficult in the beginning stages but it is bound to be because in virtually everything we do in life we are curving slightly forwards. However, without yoga's brilliant backwards bend this can easily lead to that ageing stoop. The cobra will become easier very quickly, progress at your own pace without strain. If it is very difficult for you at first, simply rest on your lower arms and elbows until your back feels better and then just progress at your own pace. Soon you won't be able to live without it!*

# 2  Pose of a cat

Watch a cat wake up and carefully stretch his spine from top to bottom by moving each vertebra in turn. This ensures that his spine is tension free and ready for action. If only the human race did the same! By practising the cat stretch, you too can release tension from your spine and really help an aching back. The movement will also tone and firm your jaw, throat, bottom, thighs and your upper arms and strengthen your wrists and hands.

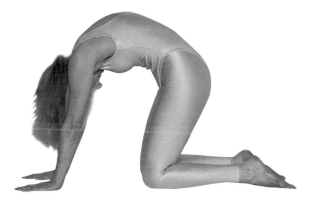

## STAGE 1

- In an all-fours position, ensure that your hands and knees are about 1 ft apart.
- Inhale deeply and arch your body like a cat in a bad mood, dropping your head in between your arms.

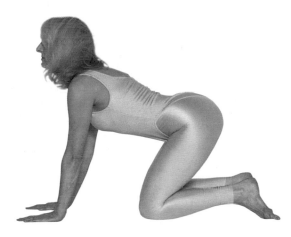

- Exhale as you lift your head and look at the ceiling, at the same time lowering your back so that your bottom sticks out.
- Repeat this sequence in slow continuous motion 5 times.

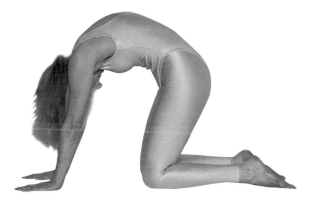

DAY TWELVE

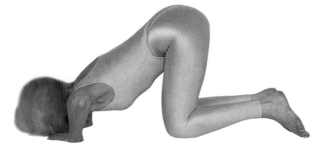

## STAGE 2

- In an all-fours position as in Stage 1, now bend your elbows and place your chin on the floor.
- Inhale and again arch your back into a hump and gently draw your right knee towards your forehead.

- Exhale, lift your head and, looking at the ceiling, lift your right leg in the air and point your toes to the ceiling.
- Repeat the sequence 3 times and then repeat with the left leg.
- Following the repetition take a deep breath in and, as you exhale gently, lower your bottom to your heels placing your forehead on the floor in front of your knees, keeping your arms at full stretch. This is called 'pose of a swan'.
- Stay in this position for a count of 10, breathing normally.
- Inhale and slowly return to an upright position, stretch your arms up above your head in a straight line with your palms together and thumbs crossed.
- Exhale and relax. There is no need to repeat the movement.

### Extra Help
*If you find Stage 2 difficult in the beginning stages, don't worry. First do Stage 1 followed by 'pose of a swan' until you feel more agile. If you do have an aching back, you will find Stage 1 a real blessing. Use it after you have finished jobs that can lead to an aching back, such as gardening.*

# 3 Alternate nostril breathing

This soothing and calming movement relieves tension that plays havoc with your skin, hair and energy flow. It is really calming. Remember, how you look on the outside is a reflection of what is going on inside, so use this whenever tension strikes.

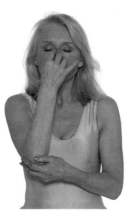

- Sit comfortably in either a crossed-leg or kneeling position or, if more convenient, your chair will do fine.
- Close your eyes.
- Place your right thumb on your right nostril, your next two fingers on the bridge of your nose and your next finger on your left nostril.
- Support your right elbow with your left hand.
- Unblock your right nostril and keeping your left one blocked inhale for a count of 5.
- Block the right nostril and keeping both nostrils closed hold your breath for a count of 5.
- Unblock your left nostril and slowly exhale for a count of 5.
- Hold your breath out for a count of 5.
- Inhale through your left nostril for a count of 5.

Continue this slow beautiful relaxing, breathing exercise for 10 rounds. It will help you relax, and cope with even the most upsetting situation and is excellent to do before going to sleep.

---

## TAKE 2 MINUTES: beauty tip

**To relieve stress –** Stress plays havoc with your looks, just as when you are stressed mole hills look like mountains and life becomes distorted. Try this simple exercise to help relieve the tension.

- Sit straight and slow down your breathing. Inhale for a count of 5, hold your breath for 5, then exhale slowly and calmly for 5. Repeat this 10 times, or simply do the alternative nostril exercise.
- Now visualize a lake but see the surface as turbulent with the wind blowing on it. Look closely at the lake and see how distorted the reflections are. Nothing looks right. This is how your mind behaves when it is stressed. Now keep your breathing slow and calm and imagine the lake also calming down. See the reflections coming back to normal and eventually see the lake so calm that the reflections are perfect. Your mind is like that beautifully calm lake, when calm and relaxed you see things perfectly clearly. Now concentrate on the beautifully calm lake and relax, relax, relax.
- Look in the mirror when you have finished this relaxation and see how much better you look!

# DAY 13

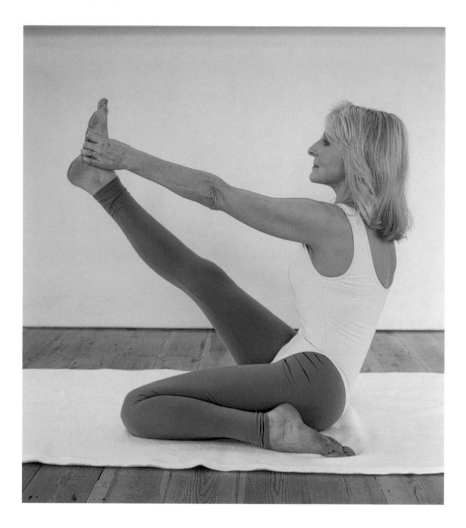

❝ *Live your life each day as you would climb a mountain. An occasional glance towards the summit keeps the goal in mind, but many beautiful scenes are to be observed from each new vantage point. Climb slowly, steadily enjoying each passing moment, and the view from the summit will serve as a fitting climax for the journey.* ❞

HAROLD B. MELCHART

## TAKE 2 MINUTES: to focus on your goals

Visualize your goals. Take a little time to reflect now on how you are feeling every day – you are doing very well and we are nearly half way, but don't wait until Day 28 to be happy. Give thanks for your health, happiness, friends and job. Add 3 more blessings to your list.

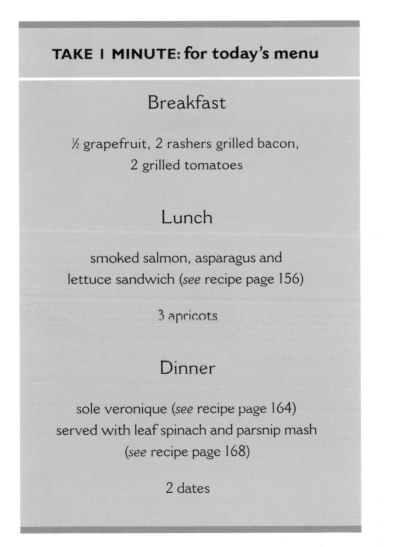

### TAKE 1 MINUTE: for today's menu

#### Breakfast

½ grapefruit, 2 rashers grilled bacon,
2 grilled tomatoes

#### Lunch

smoked salmon, asparagus and
lettuce sandwich (*see* recipe page 156)

3 apricots

#### Dinner

sole veronique (*see* recipe page 164)
served with leaf spinach and parsnip mash
(*see* recipe page 168)

2 dates

# TAKE 25 MINUTES: for today's exercises

Carefully do all the movements you have learnt this week. It will take you about 25 minutes.

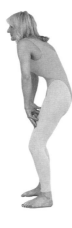

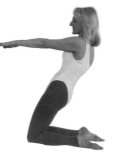

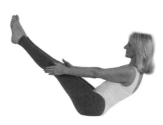

• Abdominal lift

• Tummy and thigh toner

• Pose of a boat

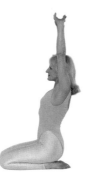

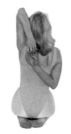

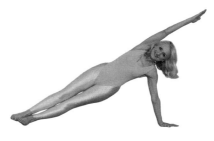

• Pose of a mountain

• Pose of a cow

• Sideways body raise

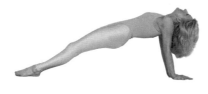

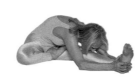

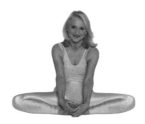

• Pose of a plane

• Alternate leg pull

• Thigh stretch

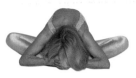

* Pose of a star

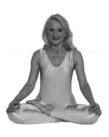

* The lotus positions

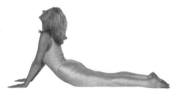

* Back stretch

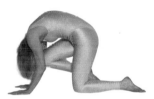

* Simple twist

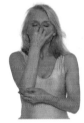

* Wide-angled leg stretch

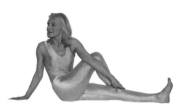

* Pose of a cobra

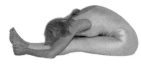

* Pose of a cat

* Alternate nostril breathing

## TAKE 2 MINUTES: beauty tip

**Stay groomed** – Even the most beautifully groomed person can suffer from a fallen hem-line, dusty shoes, spinach on their teeth, a badly chipped nail, a cut finger or laddered tights. In case of such eventualities, I keep in my make-up bag:

* 1 toothbrush (the size of a large marble – you can get them from slot machines at motorway service stations),
* 1 sachet shoe cleaner (about 1 in square, available in supermarkets),
* 2 safety pins (tiny ones are great for fixing a dropped hem),
* 1 Elastoplast (ideal for covering a chipped nail),
* 1 black felt-tipped pen (ideal for fixing scuffed heels).

I have used all of them myself in the past and also have helped friends in a crisis. If wearing tights, it is easy to find tiny rolled-up tights for travelling and well worth keeping a spare pair in your bag.

# DAY 14

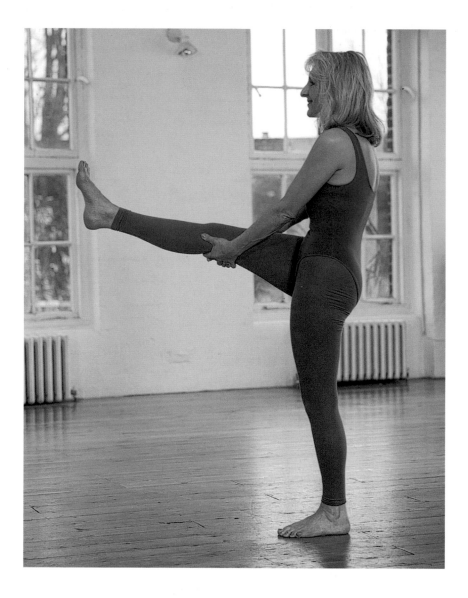

*Know what you want to do, hold the thought firmly, and do every day what should be done, and every sunset will see you much nearer the goal.*

ELBERT HUBBARD

## TAKE 2 MINUTES: to focus on your goals

Well done, you are half way there! Turn to your notebook, weigh yourself, enter in your notebook your weight and measurements. I do hope you are now feeling better and more in control. You now should have lost at least 5 lbs in weight. Well done! Right, let's continue. Focus on your goals. If you have achieved any of them tick them off and pat yourself on the back – it's nice to reward yourself with a small present – you deserve it. Set new goals if necessary.

## TAKE 1 MINUTE: for today's menu

### Breakfast

1 glass fresh orange juice, 1 slice wholegrain toast with a little butter, 1 boiled egg

### Lunch

4 oz poached salmon, 2 tsp mayonnaise with chopped chives added, green salad of rocket, watercress, endive and sprouts, 2 tsp oil and lemon juice dressing

1 peach

### Dinner

scallops with ginger and grapefruit (*see* recipe page 164), celeriac mash, fresh spinach

1 kiwi fruit

## TAKE 5 MINUTES: for today's exercises

Go for a long walk in the woods or park; see and really appreciate the flowers, trees and wildlife.

## TAKE 2 MINUTES: beauty tip

**The Lion Exercise** – This is a brilliant face lift! The movement stimulates blood flow to your face so invigorating the skin. It tones the muscles of the face and neck giving you an excellent face lift. It stimulates blood flow to the back of the throat and is a wonderful aid in helping to relieve a sore throat. By opening the eyes very wide, it tones the eye muscles and the delicate skin surrounding the eyes. This movement has excellent benefits but do it alone because it looks dreadful!

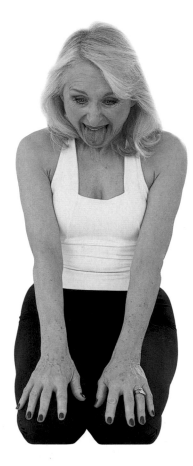

- Sit straight in a kneeling or classic crossed leg position and place your hands on your knees.

- Inhale deeply then exhale forcibly through your mouth and simultaneously stick your tongue out aiming it to curl over your chin, stretch your hands out wide and open your eyes as wide as possible. Hold for a count of 10 then inhale, relax and repeat 3 times.

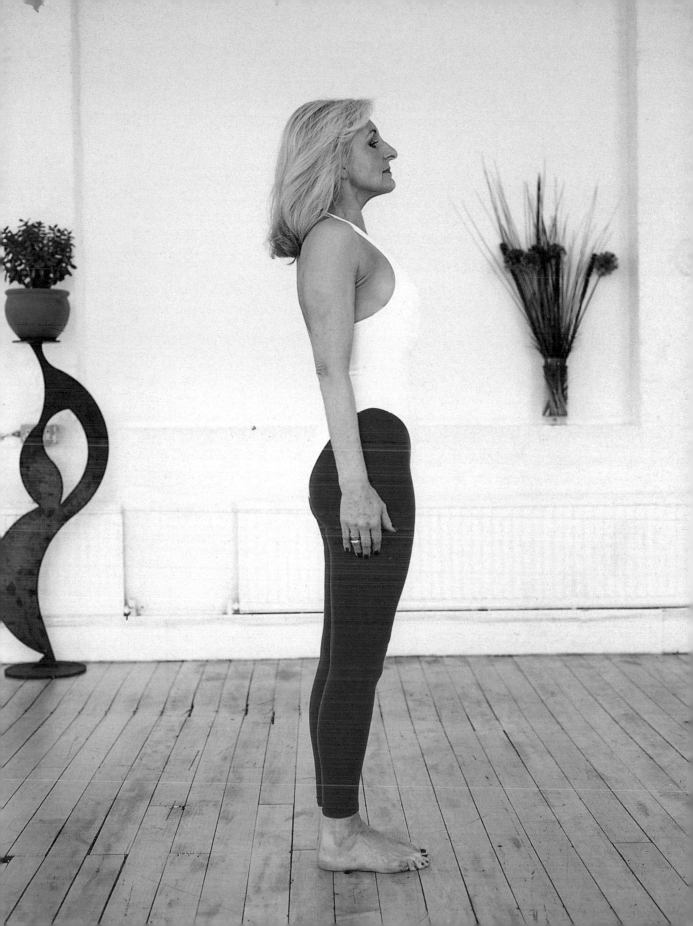

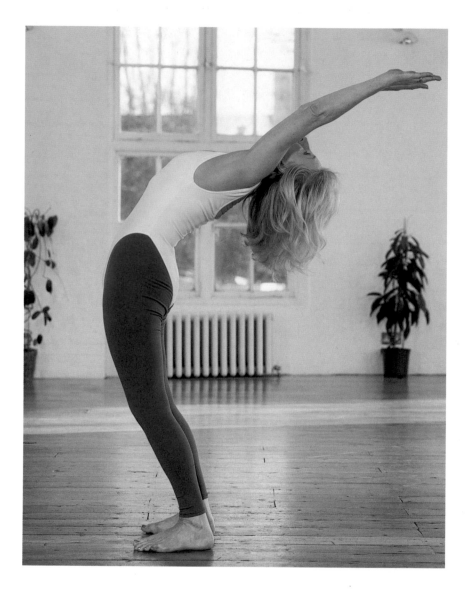

6 *Reach high, for stars lie hidden in your soul.*
*Dream deep for every dream precedes the goal.* 9
PAMELA VAULL STARR

# TAKE 2 MINUTES: to focus on your goals

We are now in Week 3. Focus on your goals – never skip this step. It is easy to think that you now know your goals so you stop reading them – this is a huge mistake. It is only by constant reading repetition that they will become lodged in your sub-conscious mind. Visualize a great day ahead, concentrate today on having a wonderful zest for life. Enjoy and put incredible enthusiasm into every project. When you pour enthusiasm into life, life will handsomely reward you.

## TAKE 1 MINUTE: for today's menu

### Breakfast

½ grapefruit, 1 poached egg,
1 slice wholegrain toast

### Lunch

4 oz parma ham, 2 figs, small portion coleslaw
(made with shredded red and white cabbage
and grated carrot) and 2 tsp mayonnaise,
small green salad with 2 tsp dressing

### Dinner

4 oz grilled halibut and lemon juice,
2 tsp tartare sauce, steamed carrots, fresh peas
with mint

10 grapes

# 1 Pose of a camel

This is one of my favourites; it opens your chest releasing tightness and as a result is a great help for asthmatics. It tones and firms your thighs, firms your jaw and throat, tones your abdominals, gives your spine tremendous flexibility and greatly releases tension.

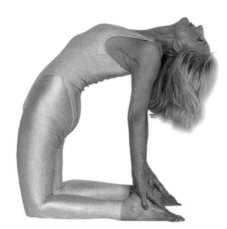

- Adopt a high kneeling position with your knees about 1 ft apart. Place your hands at your waistline with your thumbs in front and your fingers behind.
- Inhale deeply and with full lungs gently relax backwards, keeping your thighs straight and your bottom pushed forwards. Arch backwards and drop your hands, aiming the palms of your hands on your feet. (If this is not possible, and it rarely is to start with, just hold your maximum backwards stretch keeping your hands at your waistline.)
- Exhale and hold your maximum position for a count of 5, breathing normally.

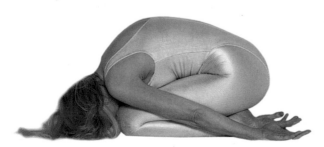

- Inhale as you return to an upright position.
- Exhale and carefully relax forwards, placing your head on the floor in front of your knees, your bottom on your heels and your arms by your sides and relax in this position known as the 'pose of a child' for a count of 5, breathing normally.
- Inhale and slowly return to an upright position. Exhale, relax and repeat.

# 2   Pose of a rabbit

**Caution:** Do not attempt if you have high blood pressure or any head or neck area problems.

This is a wonderful tension release for the neck and spine and a great help to headache sufferers. It is very beneficial to the skin and hair due to the extra circulation in that area. It stimulates the thyroid and parathyroid glands in the neck and is most beneficial to the sinuses. An excellent movement for relieving tension from the neck and stimulating blood flow to the brain.

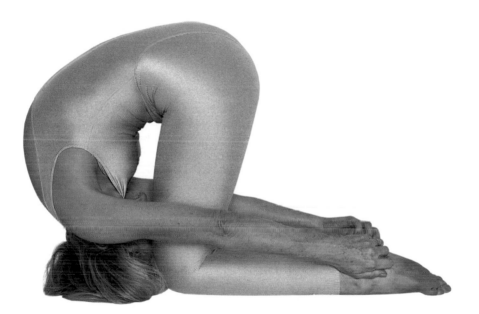

- Kneel with your bottom on your heels and place your forehead on a thick mat. Place your hands on your heels.
- Inhale and, as you exhale, place your forehead on your knees then gripping your heels firmly with your hands, gently lift your bottom in the air, aiming eventually to have your arms straight and your thighs perpendicular with the floor. To accomplish this you may have to nudge your knees gently towards your forehead and this can take a while. Don't strain – just take it carefully.

- Make sure your body weight is supported by your arms stretching back to your heels with only a fraction of it on your head.
- Hold your maximum position for a count of 8, increasing to 10 as you become better at the pose. Then inhale and slowly lower your bottom to your heels and relax in the 'pose of a child'. Hold for a count of 10, then slowly return to a sitting position and relax, lying down for a count of 10. Do not repeat.

# 3 Head and neck exercises

This movement, as well as releasing tension from the neck, can actually help remove the calcium deposits that can settle on the joint surfaces, so helping combat tightness and stiffness in the neck. It is excellent in helping to remove a double chin and it tones and firms the muscles of the jaw and throat. If you are having a hard day, it is a good idea to stop and do this movement in your office in order to relieve the build up of tension in your neck. It is really beneficial for headache and migraine sufferers, and a great tension release for 'the proverbial pain in the neck'. I have never seen as many tense and tight necks in 30 years of teaching yoga as I have in the last 3 years!

**Caution:** Please go gently with this movement making the tiniest movements to start with and only gradually increasing the movement as your neck eases. If you are having problems with your neck, then please check with your doctor before attempting this movement.

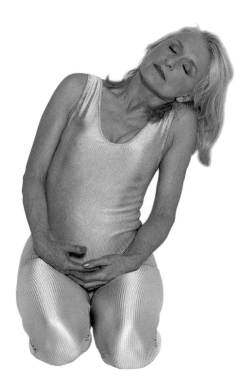

- Sit with your back straight and in either a cross-legged or kneeling position.
- Gently drop your head forwards then slowly roll it to the right, gently allow it to roll back and then let it roll slowly to the left

and then slowly and carefully forwards. Make 3 slow gentle circles to the right and then gently rotate the head the other way round making 3 circles to the left.

## TAKE 2 MINUTES: beauty tip

**Scalp massage –** To invigorate your scalp try this wonderful massage. It is best done at night before bedtime or any other time your scalp feels tense. As well as stimulating your hair follicles so encouraging beautiful shiny hair, it is also a great tension reliever.

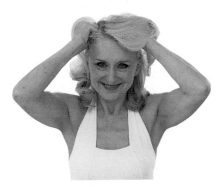

- Sit straight and place your hands in your hair near to your scalp, grab your hair and pull it very gently. While pulling it, make 3 small circles with the part that you are pulling. Then release it.

- Now find another area and repeat. Continue until your entire scalp has been stimulated.

# DAY 16

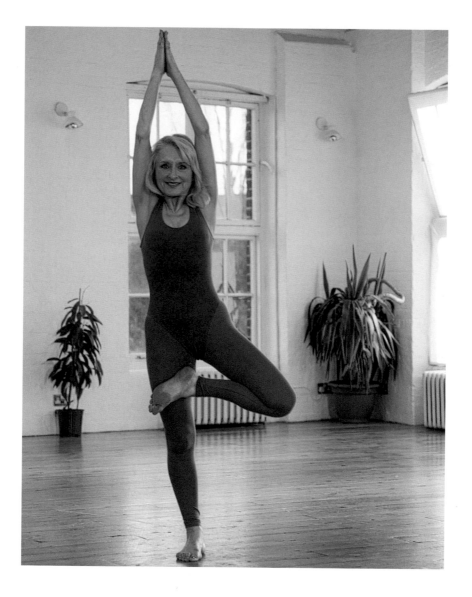

' *Dance as though no one is watching you,*
*Love as though you have never been hurt before,*
*Sing as though no one can hear you,*
*Live as though heaven is on earth.* '

SOUZA

## TAKE 2 MINUTES: to focus on your goals

Look at your goals and your statement. Focus on it and be grateful for all the blessings you possess. Add at least 3 more to your list.

As you slim, tone and beautify your body and inspire your mind, new energy is released. One great thing to do with this energy is to start to unclutter your life. Today, if you have time, try and tidy just one drawer and throw out all unnecessary items. This will really release extra energy within you.

## TAKE I MINUTE: for today's menu

### Breakfast

a pink smoothie – combine 1 natural low-fat organic yoghurt with 1 banana, a carton of blueberries and 1 tsp honey

### Lunch

grilled goat's cheese on mixed leaf salad
(*see* recipe page 157)

2 fresh figs

### Dinner

4 oz chargrilled steak and a little mustard or barbecue sauce, 2 grilled mushrooms with garlic, steamed marrow and cauliflower

2 slices fresh pineapple

# 1  Sideways leg raise

An incredible movement for ensuring the flexibility of the hips and tone of the inner thighs it is also a great help in relieving lower back tension.

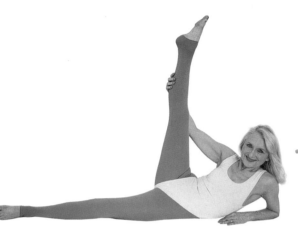

• Lie on your right side with your body in a straight line, one leg on top of the other, and prop yourself up on your right upper arm with your elbow bent and your fingertips pointing to your waist.

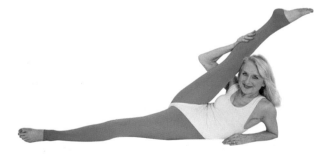

• Inhale deeply and, as you exhale, gently lift your upper leg and clasp it with your left hand. Without straining, draw it inwards towards your left ear. Hold your maximum position breathing normally for a count of 5, then gently lower your leg, relax and repeat. Perform the movement twice on the other side.

### *Extra Help*

Sometimes when starting this movement your hips may be quite painful. It can help if in the beginning stages if you bend your knee and rotate your hip forwards before carefully lifting it up without strain. With practice, the flexibility in your hips will greatly improve.

# 2   Half locust

**Caution:** Do not do this movement if pregnant

The half locust relieves lower back tension and firms and tones the bottom and thighs. It releases tension in the lower abdomen and can help to relieve constipation.

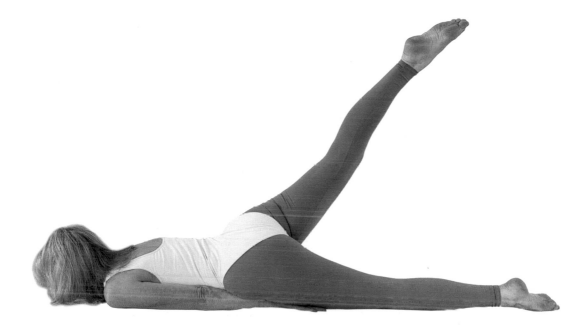

- Lie face down on your mat with your feet together and your chin on the floor. Have your hands and arms by your sides or under your thighs.
- Inhale deeply and as you exhale gently lift your right leg from the floor keeping it straight.
- Don't twist or roll over on your side.
- Hold for a count of 5, breathing normally, increasing the hold to 10 as you progress

- in the position.
- Lower your leg and relax, then repeat on the other side.
- Repeat the entire sequence twice.
- Lift your bottom in the air and stretch it back to your heels with your arms straight out in front of you into the 'pose of a swan'. Hold for a count of 10 then gently return to an upright position.

### *Extra Help*

The chief problem here is that your desire to lift your leg higher means there is a tendency to roll over to the side or bend the legs. It is much better to lift the leg just a little way to begin with, rather than getting the lop-sided habit. Remember, practice makes perfect.

# 3  Full locust

**Caution:** Do not do this movement if pregnant. If you have a weak back, read 'Extra Help' first.

This posture is a wonderful strengthener for the lower back. It tones the bottom and thighs; helps to relieve constipation and menstrual troubles and can help to relieve the pain of tennis elbow. I also heartily recommend doing three of these before bed as an aid to calm restful sleep.

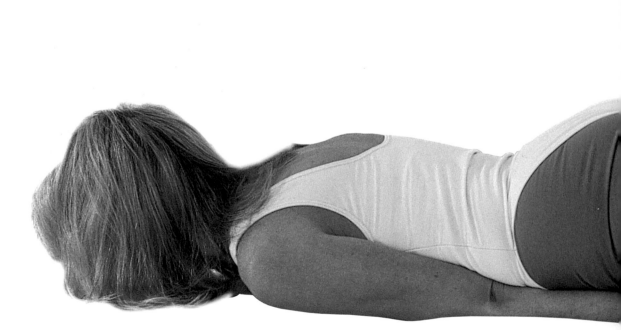

• Lie on your stomach with your chin on the floor and your arms under your body palms facing downwards and inhale deeply. As you exhale lift both legs from the floor, making sure you keep them together and straight. Hold for a count of 5, then slowly lower your legs, relax and repeat twice.

• After completing the locust posture place your hands either side at shoulder level, inhale deeply and lift your bottom in the air and stretch it gently back to your heels and remain in this posture known as 'pose of a swan' for a count of 5. This is an excellent movement to stretch out and realign the spine following the locust position.

### Extra Help

If you have a weak lower back, please ensure that you practice the half locust and feel really comfortable with it before starting the full locust and then progress with caution holding only for a count of 1 to start with, increasing to 5 as you make progress in the position.

### TAKE 2 MINUTES: beauty tip

**Walk beautifully** – This will make you look graceful and taller. Always keep your shoulders back and your head high. Walk from the hips with nice even paces, pushing your hips slightly forwards as you walk.

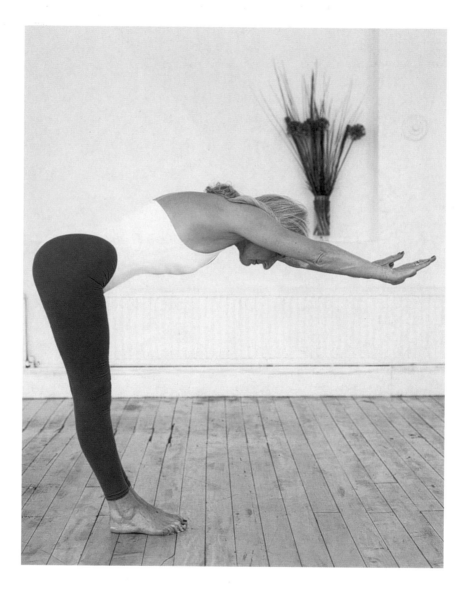

*Let us be grateful to people who make us happy;
they are the charming gardeners who make our
souls blossom.*

MARCEL PROUST

## TAKE 2 MINUTES: to focus on your goals

I do hope you are now enjoying your 10 minutes in the morning and realize it is such an important part of your day. Give thanks for all your blessings. Today focus on helping someone else to be happy, maybe do them a small good turn or pay them a compliment. Spend a little time to talk to them and be interested in what they have to say.

## TAKE 1 MINUTE: for today's menu

### Breakfast

1 tomato juice, 1 scrambled egg on
1 slice wholegrain toast

### Lunch

mixed seafood salad (*see* recipe page 157)

1 slice honeydew melon

### Dinner

Chicken with bacon and tomato sauce
(*see* recipe page 157) served with French beans

½ mango

# 1   Pose of a heron

## STAGE 1

This clever movement tones the back of your thighs and is a great help in smoothing away cellulite. It stretches out your hamstrings and is a very important component in helping to relieve lower back problems.

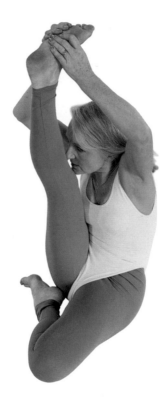

- Sit on the floor with both legs straight out in front of you.
- Place your left foot into the space between your legs resting your heel on the floor by your groin.
- Bend your right leg and interlock your hands under your right foot.
- Correct your posture, inhale deeply and as you exhale slowly aim to stretch your right leg and bring it upwards. Your eventual aim is to straighten your leg and place your knee on your chin with your back and right leg straight.
- If this is not possible (and it rarely is in the beginning stages) aim to straighten your right leg by adjusting the position of your hands to your calf or knee to enable you to do this, and then lift the leg as high as possible.
- Hold for a count of 5, breathing normally then exhale, gently lower your leg, relax and repeat on the other side.
- Repeat the entire movement.

## STAGE 2

Stage 2 is slightly stronger stretch, so please don't attempt it until you feel comfortable with stage 1.

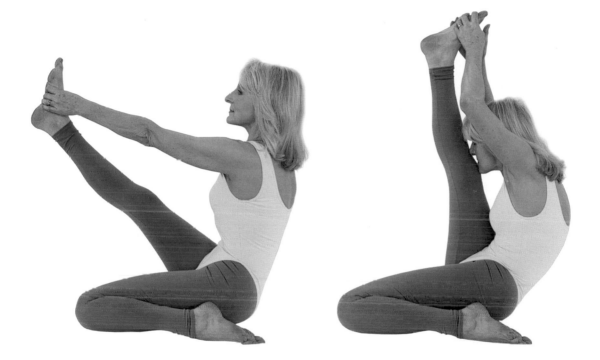

- Sitting comfortably with both legs straight out in front of you, place your left foot on the outside of your left thigh by your left buttock. Interlock your hands under your right foot and carefully straighten your right leg.

- Gently draw your right knee towards your chin. Hold your maximum position for a count of 5, gradually increasing to 10 as you progress. Gently lower your leg and repeat, then perform the movement on the other side.

### *Extra Help*

If you find it difficult to balance to begin with, place your right hand on the floor to give you support and stretch the right leg, holding it with your left hand.

# 2  Backwards bend

The backwards bend is one of my favourites. It relieves tension in the chest, firms the neck and throat, corrects poor posture and is wonderful for firming and toning the thighs. It is a great way to stretch out your tensions.

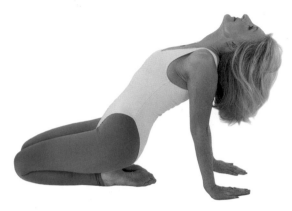

- Kneel with your bottom on your heels and place your hands on the floor behind you with your fingers pointing backwards.

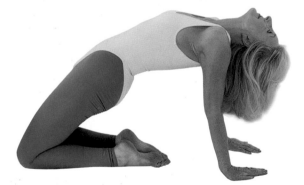

- Take a deep breath in and lift your bottom gently from your heels. Drop your head back. Exhale in your maximum position and stay in this position, breathing normally, for a count of 5, building the count up to 10 as you progress in this posture.

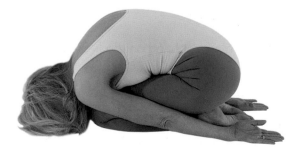

- Inhaling gently, lower your bottom to your heels. Exhale and place your hands by your side. Relax in this beautiful relaxing position, which is called 'pose of a child'. Repeat the movement once.

# 3  Pose of a monkey

You think that you will never manage this movement but with daily practice, you will – and when you do you'll feel fantastic. Mentally, it opens new horizons as you think that having mastered this seemingly difficult movement then what else is possible? Physically, it relieves lower back tension and can help sciatica sufferers. It is great for toning and firming your thighs and increasing the flexibility of your hamstrings. With your new flexibility in your lower back, your walk will look 10 years younger.

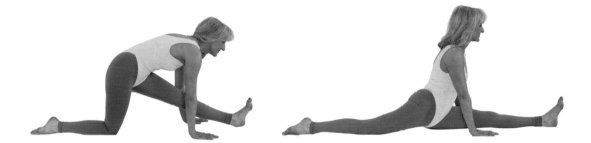

- Kneel on your mat with your knees about 1 ft apart. Place your hands on the floor in front of you, directly under your shoulders and about 1 ft apart.
- Stretch your right leg out in front of you, ensuring that your hands are either side of your right leg and are supporting your weight.

- Keeping your weight on your hands, inhale deeply and, as you exhale, stretch your right foot forwards as far as possible without strain.
- Hold your maximum position for a count of 5, then slowly draw your right leg back to a kneeling position and relax and repeat to the other side. Repeat the entire sequence once.

## Extra Help

Please don't be put off if your early attempts seem feeble. With gentle daily practice, you really will master this stretch.

### TAKE 2 MINUTES: beauty tip

**Take care of your eyes** – Your eyes, as Shakespeare wrote, are 'the windows of your soul'. It is so important to look after them.

- Tired eyes can be helped by a gentle bath. Put ¼ teaspoon full of salt into a sterilized cup containing ¼ pint of lukewarm previously boiled water. Use this solution to bathe your eyes – use a sterilized egg cup if you don't possess an eye bath.

# DAY 18

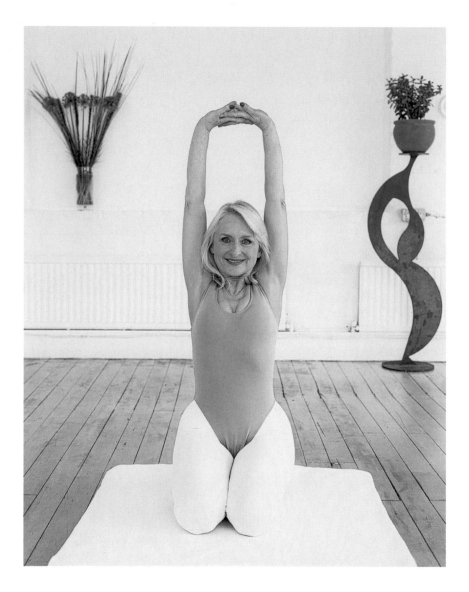

❛ *Half the things that people do not succeed in are through fear of making the attempt.* ❜
JAMES NORTHCOTE

## TAKE 2 MINUTES: to focus on your goals

Visualize a lovely day ahead. Today try to conquer fear. This can be difficult but why not just face one tiny thing that you are afraid of. Maybe you have had a good idea to make something at your place of work a little better, but you are scared of telling your boss. Just do it – all she can say is no, but most likely she will be thrilled at your suggestion and delighted that you explained it to her.

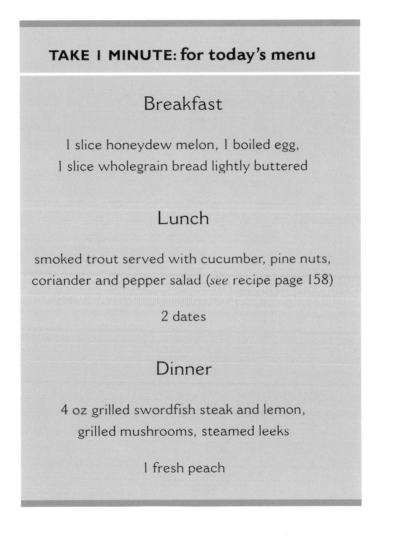

### TAKE 1 MINUTE: for today's menu

## Breakfast

1 slice honeydew melon, 1 boiled egg,
1 slice wholegrain bread lightly buttered

## Lunch

smoked trout served with cucumber, pine nuts,
coriander and pepper salad (*see* recipe page 158)

2 dates

## Dinner

4 oz grilled swordfish steak and lemon,
grilled mushrooms, steamed leeks

1 fresh peach

# 1 Pose of a dog

It's difficult to express adequately the benefits of this brilliant movement. It increases the flexibility of the spine, stretches the hamstrings and calf muscles and can even help get rid of calciferous spurs on the heels. It strengthens and tones the arms, relieves tension in the wrist, lower back, neck and shoulders. It is excellent for helping to prevent menstrual cramps and lower backache. It tones the liver, spleen and kidneys, firms the jaw and throat and is a wonderful toner for your bottom and thighs.

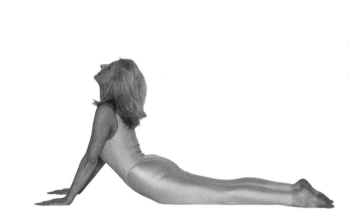

- Lie face down on your mat and place your hands either side of you in line with your shoulders with your fingertips facing forwards. Place your forehead on the floor.
- Take a deep breath in, as you exhale place your chin on the floor.
- Inhale and keeping your lower abdomen on the floor slowly lift your upper body from the floor into 'pose of a cobra' (*see* page 64). Stretch into the movement as far as you can without strain, drop your head back and relax in your maximum position. Exhale and hold for a count of 5, breathing normally.

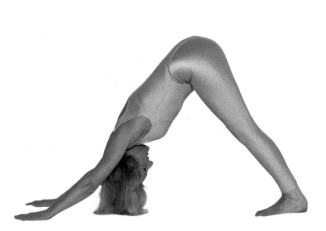

- Inhale deeply and as you exhale tuck your toes under and, pushing down hard on your hands, lift your bottom in the air and aim to stretch your heels to the floor drawing your head down between your arms so that your body resembles an inverted 'v'. Hold this position for a count of 5, then slowly swing your head back between your arms, bend your elbows and gently lower your body to the floor. Relax and repeat once to start with but, as your strength, ability and agility improve, increase to 3 repeats.

## 2  Full twist

The twist is wonderful for releasing tension in the entire spine and giving it amazing flexibility. It stimulates extra blood flow to the spinal nerves. It increases flexibility in the lower back, hips and shoulders, slims the midriff and waistline and hips, and firms the neck, jaw and throat.

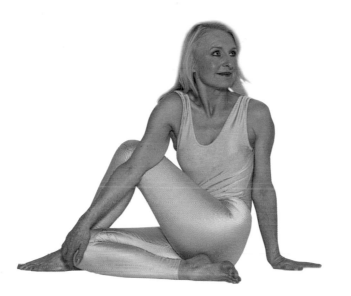

- Sit up straight with both legs straight out in front of you and place your right foot in the middle between your legs with your heel by your groin.
- Inhale and bring your left foot over your right thigh and place your left heel on the floor on the outer side of your right thigh.
- Exhale and place your left hand on the floor behind your back.
- Take a deep breath and, as you exhale, take

your right arm on the outside of the left knee and place it on the right knee.
- Inhale deeply and, as you exhale, carefully rotate your body and turn your head over your left shoulder. Hold this position for a count of 5, breathing normally, increasing to 10 as you progress in the movement.
- Slowly inhale and return your body to face the front, exhale, relax and repeat on the other side. Then repeat the entire movement.

# 3   The plough

**Caution:** Do not attempt this movement if you have high blood pressure or any head or neck area problems. Do not do this movement if you are pregnant.

An amazing movement – it releases tension in the lower back and can help to relieve backache. It stimulates extra blood to the thyroid and parathyroid glands in the neck, helping to keep them in excellent condition. This beautifully relaxing movement stretches out the spine, stimulates blood flow to the head and neck area so helping your skin, hair and brain cells.

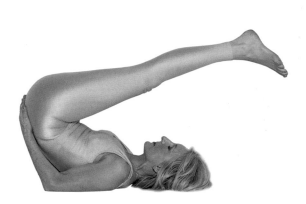 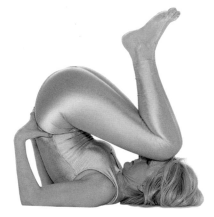

## STAGE 1

- Lie down with your back on your mat. Inhale and bend your knees and gently lift your bottom as far as you can from the floor but make sure that you don't strain.
- Place your hands on your lower back to give support and aim to have your legs parallel to the floor. This is stage 1 of the plough. Hold this movement for just 10 seconds in the beginning, building up very gradually until

you are able to stay in the position for 30 seconds.
- Gently draw your knees to your forehead and very slowly roll down your spine just a vertebra at a time until your bottom touches the floor. Interlock your hands around your knees, then gently rock from side to side relaxing your back into the floor. Lie down on your back, breathe slowly and deeply and relax.

*Our plans miscarry because they have not aim.*
*When a man does not know what harbour he is making*
*for no wind is the right wind.*

SENECA

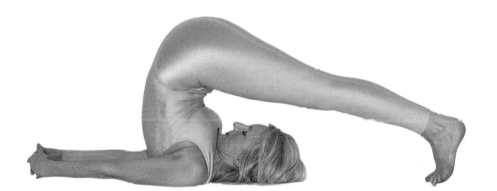

## STAGE 2

- As you progress in the plough, you will find that the movement eases tension in your lower back and your feet will eventually touch the floor. When this happens, you no longer need your hands to support your back, so stretch them in the opposite direction to your feet, interlock them and enjoy the lovely stretch. Hold the position for 30 seconds, breathing normally, and then support your back and roll down exactly as in stage 1. Note that as you progress in this movement, a longer stay in it is a wonderful stress reliever. Build up gently to a longer hold. I recommend increasing the hold by 30 seconds a week until you are able to hold it for up to 3 minutes.

### TAKE 2 MINUTES: beauty tip

**Forehead smoother –** This is a lovely tension reliever and you can see the results immediately. It is ideal to do when you are worried, hassled or over worked.

- Sit straight and close your eyes and place your fingers interleaved on the centre of your forehead.
- Take a deep breath and as you exhale slowly for a count of 7, draw your fingers slowly towards your hairline. Repeat 5 times, then look in the mirror. Don't you look calmer and more serene?

# DAY 19

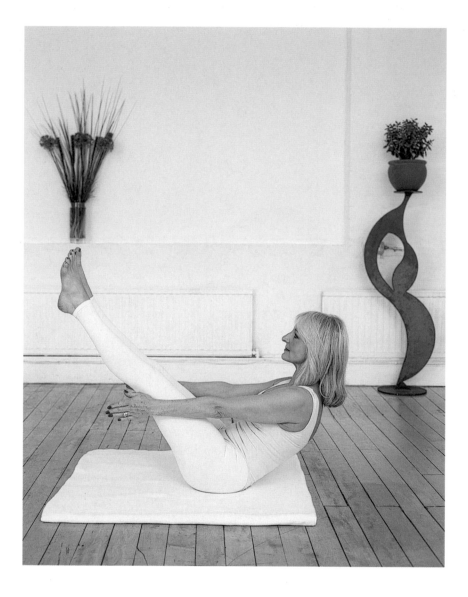

❝ *The human spirit is stronger than anything*
*that can happen to it.* ❞
GEORGE C. SCOTT

## TAKE 2 MINUTES: to focus on your goals

Focus on your beautiful healthy body goal and any other goal you have set yourself. Give thanks for your many blessings and add to your already growing list – I hope you get to 30! That may seem an incredible number but it's not really. Today, focus on trying to conquer *worry* – this great big monster can affect your health, your life, your relationships and your ability to achieve your goals. It certainly is not easy, but I find the following help tremendously.

- Focus on the outcome you desire in any worrying situation.
- Live a day at a time, forget yesterday and tomorrow and concentrate on making today a good day.
- Keep busy as most of our worries occur when we have finished work.
- Think about the worst that can happen and accept it, then do your utmost to work and prevent it happening.
- Remember most of our worries never ever happen.
- Remember there is enough power inside you to cope with anything that might happen to you.

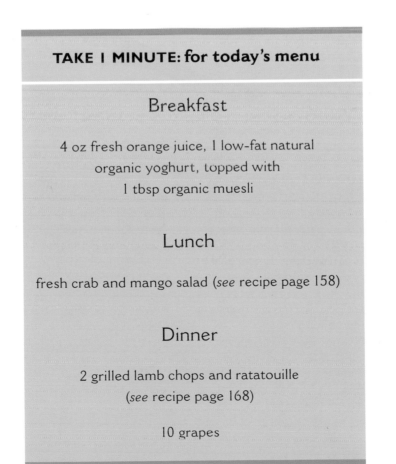

## TAKE 1 MINUTE: for today's menu

### Breakfast

4 oz fresh orange juice, 1 low-fat natural
organic yoghurt, topped with
1 tbsp organic muesli

### Lunch

fresh crab and mango salad (*see* recipe page 158)

### Dinner

2 grilled lamb chops and ratatouille
(*see* recipe page 168)

10 grapes

# 1   Maltese cross

This movement is most beneficial for relieving stiffness and pain in the hip joint and for helping people with sciatica. It tones and firms both the inner and outer thigh and releases tension in the lower back.

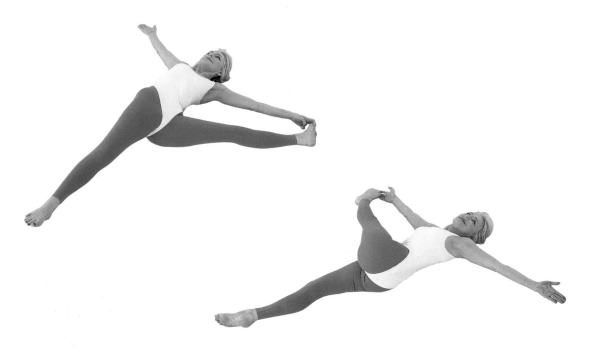

## STAGE 1

- Lie flat on your back with your arms stretched out at shoulder level and your legs together so that you resemble a cross.
- Inhale and, as you exhale, keeping your left heel on the floor, slowly stretch your left leg and gradually aim your left big toe to your left hand. Your aim is to clasp your big toe! (This sounds incredibly easy but the heel must not leave the floor and don't worry if at first only a small movement is possible. You will improve very quickly in this position.)
- Hold your maximum stretch without strain for a count of 5, then slowly draw the leg back and place it in the starting position close to the other one.
- Repeat the movement to the right and then perform the entire sequence twice.

## STAGE 2

- Lie flat on your back with your legs together and arms palms uppermost at shoulder level.
- Inhale deeply and as you exhale, gently lift your left leg in the air and, keeping both legs straight, aim the left big toe to the centre of the right hand. Hold your maximum position for a count of 5, then inhale and carefully lift the left leg straight up in the air, then exhale as you slowly lower it to its starting position. Repeat on the other side and then repeat the entire sequence twice.

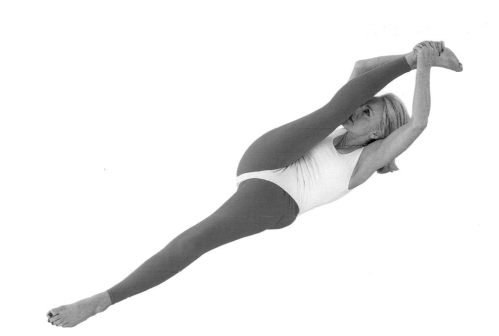

## STAGE 3

- Lie flat on your back with your arms straight and stretched out on the floor behind your head, your legs straight and together.
- Take a deep breath in and, as you exhale, lift your right leg in the air.
- Slowly lift your upper body and try to take hold of your leg, ensuring that the right leg remains straight. Your aim is to clasp your right big toe and aim the right knee to the right nostril. This is rarely possible in the beginning stages, so clasp the leg wherever you can with ease and gently draw your leg towards your head as far as possible. Ensure that both legs remain straight. Hold the clasp for a count of 5, then slowly lower both the arms and leg back to their starting position and relax. Repeat this movement to the other side and then repeat the entire sequence twice.

## TAKE 2 MINUTES: beauty tip

**Tips for beautiful hands** – To help prevent rough hands, massage your hands and nails after cooking with a little olive oil and wipe off the surplus. For redness, simply rub the juice and flesh of a fresh lemon over the hands. This is also excellent for removing fish and garlic smells from your hands. Before doing dirty jobs such as gardening, wash your hands and dry them; then dig your nails into a bar of soft soap so that the soap fills your nails. Apply hand cream and then your gardening gloves. When you have finished gardening, remove your gloves, wash your hands and apply more hand cream. This helps prevent your nails from becoming steeped in the dirt that seems to get into gardening gloves. Keep a bottle of hand cream by the bowl wherever you wash your hands, and keep a tiny bottle and a nail file in your bag for emergency use.

# DAY 20

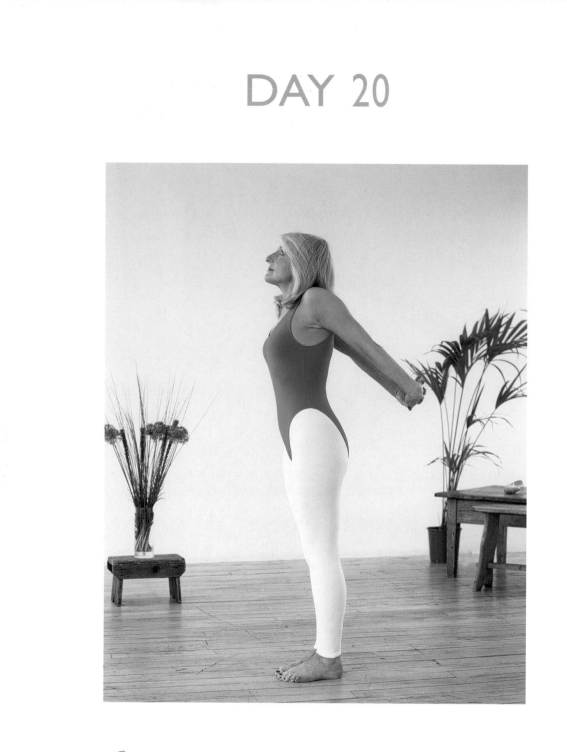

6 *Deep within man dwell those slumbering powers,*
*powers that would astonish him, that he never*
*dreamed of possessing, forces that would revolutionize*
*his life if aroused and put into action.* 9

ORISON SWETT MARSDEN

# TAKE 2 MINUTES: to focus on your goals

Focus on your goals and give thanks for your blessings. I'm glad that you have stayed with the plan so far. I hope that you are enjoying the huge benefits of your daily 10 minutes, focusing on your goals, planning a good day, doing your exercises, eating for health and vitality.

As you plan and work on your goals you will find huge power inside yourself that you never dreamed you possessed. This is incredibly exciting, so use it and amaze yourself how great you are.

## TAKE 1 MINUTE: for today's menu

### Breakfast

½ papaya and a squeeze of lime,
1 slice wholegrain toast with a little butter

### Lunch

4 oz poached salmon with 2 tsp natural
yoghurt mixed with chopped chives,
small green salad with oil and lemon juice,
small portion red coleslaw (*see* recipe page 159)

1 orange

### Dinner

beef hotpot (*see* recipe page 167),
celeriac mash

2 fresh figs

# TAKE 25 MINUTES: for today's exercises

Go through all the movements that you have learnt this week. It will take you about 25 minutes.

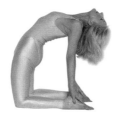

- Pose of a camel

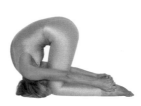

- Pose of a rabbit

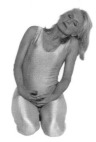

- Head and neck exercises

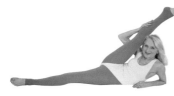

- Sideways leg raise

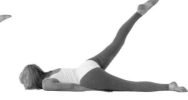

- Half locust

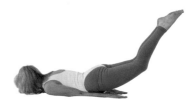

- Full locust

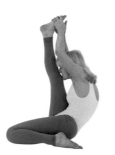

- Pose of a heron

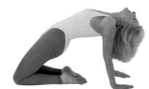

- Backwards bend

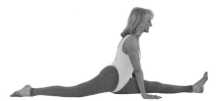

- Pose of a monkey

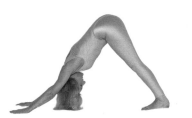

• Pose of a dog

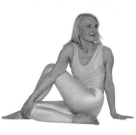

• Full twist

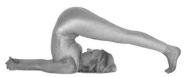

• The plough

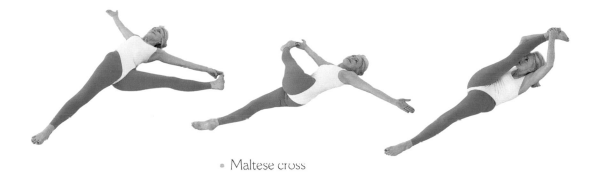

• Maltese cross

## TAKE 2 MINUTES: beauty tip

**Sleep without a pillow** – This tip was given to me over 30 years ago when I thought pillows were essential, but I'm so glad that I got rid of my pillow then. Now, at the age of 62, I don't have a double chin and I wake up feeling great in the mornings. Sit straight and lift your right arm in the air and let your left hand drop down by your side and count to 10 slowly. Now lower your right arm, place the backs of your hands together and look at the difference in colour.

This is the effect of gravity on the body and, to a small extent, this is what happens while we sleep. If your head is on a pile of pillows, your heart which is obviously below your head will not pump as much blood to the brain as when you sleep flat. By sleeping flat, your brain is adequately nourished but also you are preventing facial puffiness, bags under your eyes and a stoop.

I think I regard this as the best beauty tip I was given. Don't try to sleep flat immediately, especially if you have been used to 2 or 3 pillows – cut down very gently and slowly, taking about 3 months before you sleep totally flat.

# DAY 21

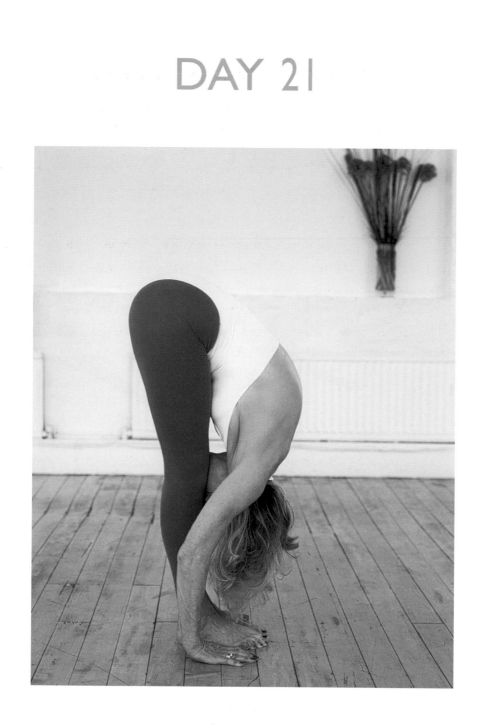

❛ *If one advances confidently in the direction of his dreams and endeavours to live the life which he has imagined, he will meet with success unexpected in common hours.* ❜

HENRY DAVID THOREAU

# TAKE 2 MINUTES: to focus on your goals

It is the end of Week 3, so it is time again to weigh yourself and take your measurements. I hope you are loving your new slimmer shape! Congratulate yourself on your achievements. Now visualize your goals again and count your blessings, and try to add some new ones to your list. Don't give up as you have only one more week to complete. Continue to put effort into your visualization, seeing yourself feeling and looking so much better and being the person you want to be.

At about this stage it is not unusual to meet some negativity from your friends and comments such as: 'Don't you get any thinner or your face will look scraggy', or well-meaning friends who try to tempt you with chocolate. This negative sort of thing will happen with any goal in life you decide to pursue. This is why we need these goals; we need to decide we are going to achieve them and have the grit and determination to go for it.

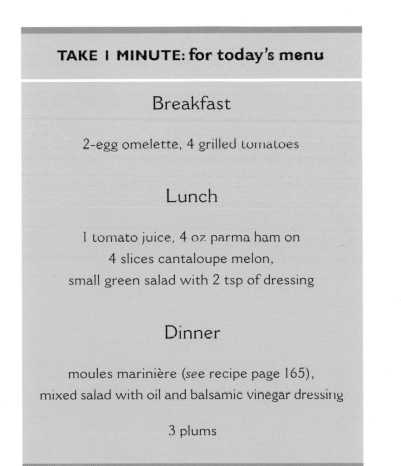

## TAKE 1 MINUTE: for today's menu

### Breakfast

2-egg omelette, 4 grilled tomatoes

### Lunch

1 tomato juice, 4 oz parma ham on
4 slices cantaloupe melon,
small green salad with 2 tsp of dressing

### Dinner

moules marinière (*see* recipe page 165),
mixed salad with oil and balsamic vinegar dressing

3 plums

# TAKE 30 MINUTES: for today's exercises

Today, go for a really long walk, breathing slowly and deeply as you walk so you feel and look glowing when you return.

## TAKE 2 MINUTES: beauty tip

**Flying high** – Have a wonderful flight on long-haul destinations by taking the following advice:

- On board make sure you are comfortable. Don't wear anything tight or restrictive. Take your shoes off and replace with warm socks and have a sweater or pashmina to hand.

- Make sure you have a really good book.

- Take off any make-up and apply your favourite moisturizer, eye cream and hand cream.

- Keep a 2-litre bottle of water with you and make sure you drink all of it during an 8-hour flight.

- Set your watch to the time of your destination.

- Every hour, if you are awake, circle your feet round to the right 3 times then to the left 3 times or write the alphabet with each foot in blocks of 8 letters each hour with each foot.

- Don't drink any alcohol and eat sparingly.

- If it is a night flight, try to sleep as much as possible.

- Before landing, cleanse and moisturize your face, clean your teeth, brush your hair, apply new make-up.

- Enjoy a light breakfast with a good cup of tea or coffee.

- On arrival keep busy, don't have a rest but stay up and then have a really early night.

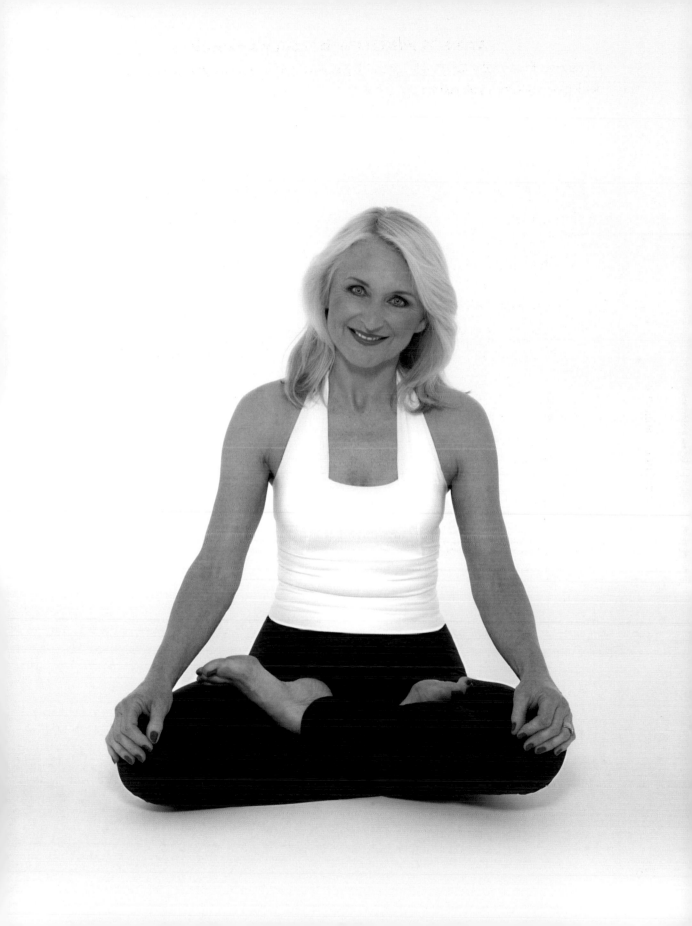

# DAY 22

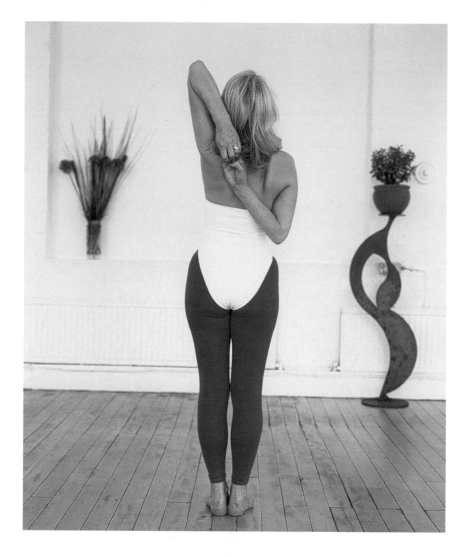

❝ *Thoughts are things that have tremendous power. Thoughts of doubt and fear are pathways to failure. When you conquer negative attitudes of doubt and fear you conquer failure. Thoughts crystallize into habit and habit solidifies into circumstance.* ❞

BRIAN ADAMS

## TAKE 2 MINUTES: to focus on your goals

Focus on your goals, visualize your lovely new body. Re-read your formula and your diet plan and count your blessings, adding 5 more to you list. Dieting is a problem for all of us and while it is always easy to quit, by now you have probably cheated a little bit – you're only human! That's OK, the wonderful thing is that you have got this far. With anything in life there are off days and people out there are always trying to make you fail. This is exactly why I have insisted you read your goals every day and visualize them. This will keep your attention focused on your goals and gradually your new eating plan will not just be a 28-day plan but become a lifelong slim habit.

## TAKE 1 MINUTE: for today's menu

### Breakfast

4 oz glass tomato juice, 1 boiled egg,
1 slice wholegrain bread with a little butter

### Lunch

chicken waldorf salad (*see* recipe page 159)

### Dinner

4 oz grilled halibut topped with 2 tsp of
Greek yoghurt mixed with 1 tsp chopped chives,
mashed parsnips, French beans

1 slice cantaloupe melon

# 1   The triangle

This incredible yoga sequence works virtually every muscle, tendon, joint and internal organ in the body. It tones and firms the hips, thighs, waistline and arms. It revitalizes the spine and helps correct lower back tension and stiffness.

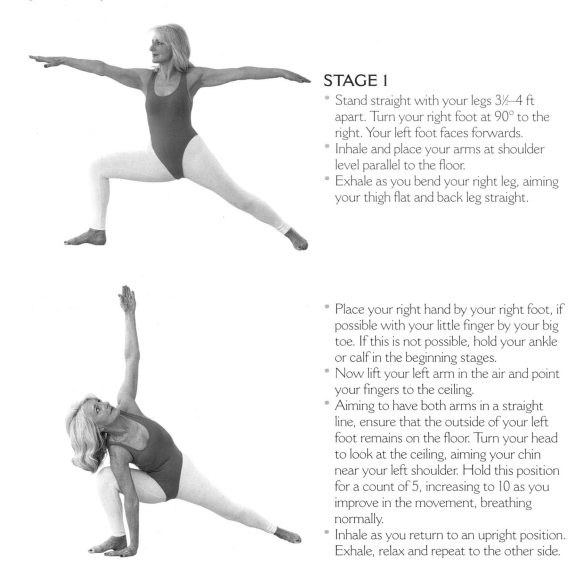

### STAGE 1

* Stand straight with your legs 3½–4 ft apart. Turn your right foot at 90° to the right. Your left foot faces forwards.
* Inhale and place your arms at shoulder level parallel to the floor.
* Exhale as you bend your right leg, aiming your thigh flat and back leg straight.

* Place your right hand by your right foot, if possible with your little finger by your big toe. If this is not possible, hold your ankle or calf in the beginning stages.
* Now lift your left arm in the air and point your fingers to the ceiling.
* Aiming to have both arms in a straight line, ensure that the outside of your left foot remains on the floor. Turn your head to look at the ceiling, aiming your chin near your left shoulder. Hold this position for a count of 5, increasing to 10 as you improve in the movement, breathing normally.
* Inhale as you return to an upright position. Exhale, relax and repeat to the other side.

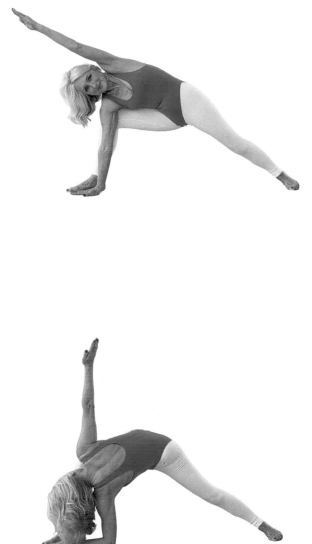

## STAGE 2

* Stand as above, with your legs 3½–4 ft apart and your right foot turned at 90° to the right and your left foot facing forwards, arms parallel to the floor at shoulder level.
* Inhale deeply and, as you exhale, bend your right knee aiming your thigh flat and back leg straight and aim to place your right thumb by your right little toe.
* Place your left arm along side your left ear in a straight line with your left foot. Hold for a count of 5, increasing to 10 as the movement becomes easier.
* Inhale and return to an upright position. Exhale, relax and repeat to the left side.

## STAGE 3

* With your legs 3½–4 ft apart, arms parallel to the floor, right foot at 90° to the right and left foot facing forwards, take a deep breath in and change your arms over so that your left arm faces over your right leg.
* Inhale and, bending your right leg, aim to have your thigh flat, place your left hand by your right foot with your left thumb by your right big toe. Gently lift your right arm in the air and rotate your torso so that you are looking at your right hand. Hold for a count of 5, breathing normally, increasing to 10 as you improve in the movement, and then slowly return to an upright position. Exhale, lower your arms and relax. Repeat to the left side, then repeat the entire triangle sequence.

### Extra Help

*Although the triangle is such a brilliant movement it is frequently a nightmare to start with. There is no easy way to do these positions – we have all had to come to terms with our own stiffness in different regions of our bodies. All I can say is persevere, follow the directions, don't strain and eventually you will love these movements and the incredible benefits that they will give you.*

# 2   Dancer's posture

This is one of yoga's most beautiful movements. As well as helping your concentration and balance, it relieves tension in your lower back, lifts and firms your bottom, and tones your thighs whilst strengthening the supporting leg.

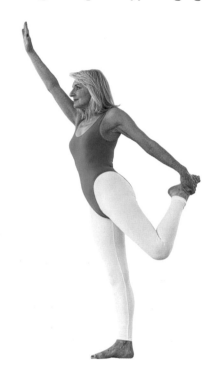

* With your feet together and with perfect posture, lift your right hand in the air, concentrate on a spot in front of you and inhale.

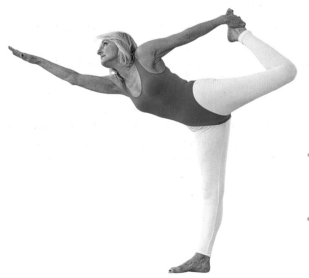

* As you exhale, grab your left foot in your left hand behind your back, and gently lift the leg as high as possible. Hold for a count of 5, breathing normally.
* Gently lower your leg and relax. Repeat to the other side and gradually increase the hold to 10 as you progress in the movement. Repeat the entire movement.

# 3 Big toe balance

This is wonderful for toning and firming the back of your thighs. It is a great help in getting rid of cellulite. It helps your coordination and balance, and releases tension in the hips and lower back.

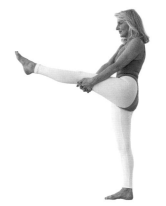 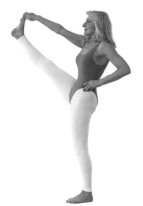

- Standing straight with both feet together, place your right hand on your right hip. Inhale and grab your left big toe in your left hand. If this is too difficult at first, don't worry. Just place both your hands under your left knee.
- Concentrating on a spot in front of you as you exhale, try to straighten your left leg, ensuring that your right leg is perfectly straight. This is difficult at first, but persevere. It is well worth it. Eventually the leg will straighten.
- Hold your maximum stretch for a count of 5, increasing to 10 as you progress in the movement. Gently lower your leg to standing position, relax and repeat to the other side. Repeat the entire sequence.

## TAKE 2 MINUTES: beauty tip

**'Wear it with an air'** – One of the most elegant women I have ever met was my mother's friend Joan. Joan adored clothes and was brilliant at watching styles and altering her clothes to give them the latest look. However, she had a very small budget. One morning she popped in to see us while my mother was bemoaning the fact that she had nothing to wear for a forthcoming event. Joan immediately helped her with her choice and when my mother tried on the clothes she looked doubtfully at her reflection in the mirror. Joan told her to just 'wear it with an air'. I've always remembered that valuable piece of advice. If you wear your clothes as though you were perfectly dressed for the occasion, you exude that feeling of confidence. Once you have dressed, forget yourself and set out to enjoy yourself instead of worrying about your outfit. So get dressed, walk tall, smile and 'wear it with an air' and you will look like the best-dressed woman in the room.

# DAY 23

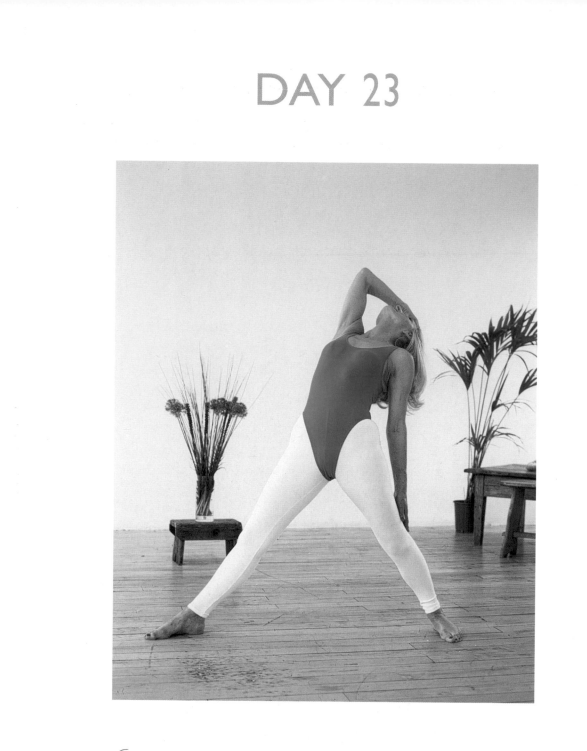

❝ *The will to win, the desire to succeed, the urge to reach your full potential; these are the keys to unlock the door to personal excellence.* ❞

EDDIE ROBINSON

## TAKE 2 MINUTES: to focus on your goals

Focus on your goals. Visualize your new shape and body and your other goals. If you have reached one of your goals tick it off and reward yourself with a small treat. Write it in your notebook and look at your list, review your goals and, if you wish, add more. Count your blessings and add at least 3 new ones to your growing list of blessings.

> *It's not happiness that makes us grateful but gratefulness that makes us happy.*

BROTHER DAVID STENDAHL RAST

## TAKE 1 MINUTE: for today's menu

### Breakfast

½ melon filled with blackberries topped with
1tbsp natural organic yoghurt

### Lunch

Egg and cress (or salad sprout) sandwich made
with 2 slices wholegrain bread filled with
1 hard-boiled egg, 2 tsp mayonnaise and
small amount of cress (or sprouts)

½ banana

### Dinner

4 oz roast chicken with fresh mixed herbs,
1 tsp cranberry sauce, 4 slices roast parsnips,
spring greens, 1 tbsp gravy

1 bowl strawberries

# 1   Head to knee balance

This movement tones and firms the thighs and bottom, and helps restore balance and relieve tension in the lower back. It stimulates blood flow to the head and neck area, and helps boost the condition of the skin and hair.

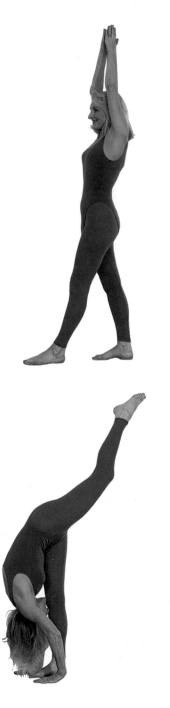

- With your feet together, lift your arms in the air and place the palms of the hands together, and cross your thumbs.
- Inhaling, place your right foot about 2 ft in front of your left foot. As you exhale, stretch carefully forwards aiming your hands to the floor either side of your right foot. In the beginning stages, you may have to bend your left knee to enable you to do this.
- Gently lift your left leg in the air, eventually aiming to point your toe towards the ceiling. Relax in the position, breathing normally, and hold for a count of 5. Then slowly inhale and lower your left leg.
- Now, with your hands flat on the floor by your right foot, aim to carefully straighten your legs. Don't strain – just persevere!
- Inhale as you lift your head, then your arms and carefully return to an upright position. Stretch your entire body, then exhale and relax.
- Repeat to the other side and notice if you find one side easier than the other – this is very important and can be caused by poor posture and imbalanced sports (such as tennis and golf). Happily, in time, yoga will correct this for you. Repeat the entire movement.
- Finally, after the last position in your maximum forwards bend, place your feet together and gently aim your chin to just below your knees. Inhale and return to a standing position, stretch your arms above your head. Exhale and relax.

# 2   Eagle balance

This is frequently a nightmare to start with – it is difficult to balance, your joints just don't seem to fit together, and your arms won't entwine. We have all started like this but, again, persevere. You will be delighted at your new flexibility. Yoga is like an oil-can, carefully increasing the flexibility of all your joints in one go. It tones your upper thighs, helps your concentration and balance, relieves tension in your lower back and stimulates blood flow to the lower abdominal organs. None of us realize how quickly our joints can stiffen – but this wonderful movement will really help!

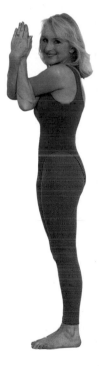

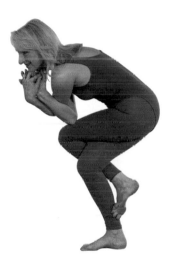

- Standing straight with your feet together, stretch both arms straight out in front of you.
- Inhale as you cross your right upper arm over your left upper arm, bend the elbows and place both hands in prayer with the thumbs together in line with your nose. Don't worry if your hands don't fit to start with, they will when flexibility is restored.

- Exhale as you repeat this with your legs. Cross the right thigh over the left, and bending the left leg entwine the right foot around the left calf, eventually aiming all 5 toes around the calf.
- Now place your chin on your upper hand, your elbow on your upper knee and hold this amazing balance for a count of 5, breathing normally while concentrating at a spot on the floor.
- Inhale as you come out of the position. Stand straight, exhale, relax and repeat on the other side. Repeat the entire movement.

# 3   Standing stick balance

This beautiful movement streamlines your body, firms and tones your bottom, thighs and calves, as well as strengthening them. It will tone and firm your upper arms and shoulders and is a fantastic tension releaser for your entire body.

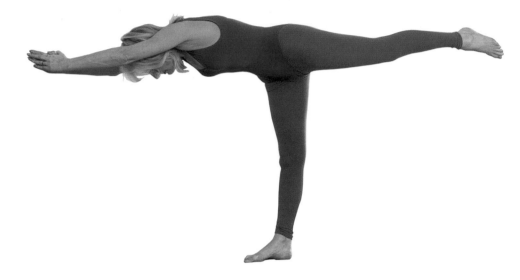

- Stand straight with your feet together and your arms up above your head, hands together and thumbs crossed.
- Inhale deeply and place your right foot 3 ft in front of your left one and concentrate on a spot to enable you to balance.
- As you exhale, gently stretch forwards placing your weight on your right leg and your left leg from the floor. Keep stretching forwards so that your arms are parallel to the floor and your head stays between your arms. Your left leg is lifted from the floor, again parallel to the floor, so that your

entire body is stretched and resembles a capital 'T'.
- Hold this position for a count of 5, breathing normally, and keep stretching whilst in the position, increasing the hold to 10 as your strength increases.
- Inhale and slowly lower your left leg to the floor placing your feet together. Gently lift your arms up above your head and stretch your entire body upwards in a perfect straight line from top to toe.
- Relax and repeat on the other side then repeat the entire balance.

### Extra Help
*At first, it isn't easy even to stand straight with your head between your straight arms and your thumbs crossed and your hands together. But doing this and concentrating on your posture in this position makes such a difference. Try doing it in front of a full-length mirror and you will see your imbalances. Daily practice of this movement will do wonders to correct your posture. In the movement, it is hard to make the arms and legs level but this will become easy as you learn to juxtaposition your body.*

# TAKE 2 MINUTES: lifestyle tip

**Sorting out your priorities** – These days we are all so busy that it is not always easy to get our priorities right. This little story will help.

'A professor was trying to explain priorities to his pupils so he gave each one of them a large glass bowl. He also gave them six large rocks, a handful of pebbles, a handful of gravel and a small bag of sand. He asked his pupils to fit all the rocks, pebbles, gravel and sand into the glass bowl. The pupils tried many ways of doing this, first placing a little sand in the bowl, then a few pebbles, then a rock etc, but try as they might, none of the pupils managed to fit all the items into a bowl.

'The professor said let this be a lesson to you, the rocks are your priorities so always attend to them first, and so he placed the rocks into the bowl. He said next come the things that are less important but never the less still things you would like to accomplish. These are represented by the pebbles. He added them next. The gravel he said represented the odds and ends that fill out lives and so he sprinkled the gravel around the rocks and pebbles. Finally, he said the sand is the stuff that can be fitted in when everything else has been accomplished and he sprinkled the sand into the cracks between rocks, pebbles and gravel and everything fitted perfectly.

'He went on to say that most people do the unnecessary items (the sand) first, and never have enough time for their real priorities, but if everyday the most important tasks are accomplished first we are well on the way to achieving our goals in life without the feeling of being overwhelmed and hassled by having too much to do.'

# DAY 24

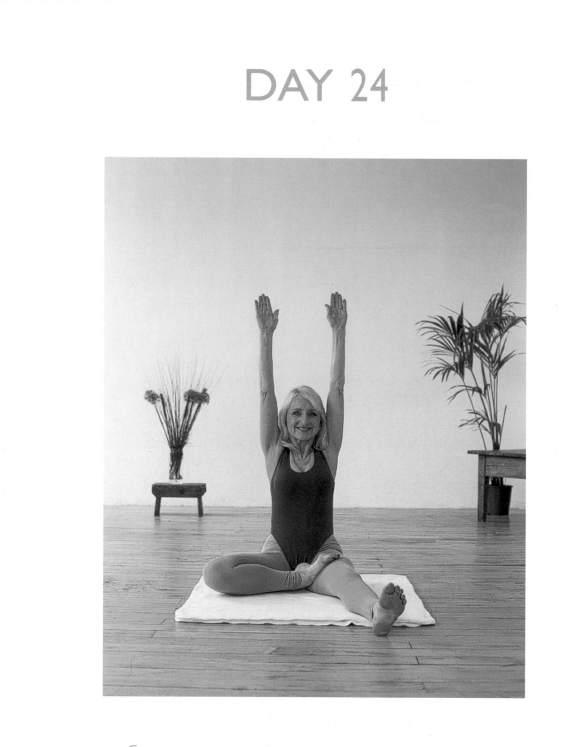

' *He turns not back who is bound to a star.* '
LEONARDO DA VINCI

## TAKE 2 MINUTES: to focus on your goals

Focus on your goals. Maybe today you are wondering that you now know your goals, whether it is really necessary to keep reading them through. I promise you that it is. This daily 10 minutes in the morning is for focusing and planning your way to your goals in life.

Count your blessings, add 3 more to your list and again give thanks for the many blessings you possess.

6 *If you count all your assets you always show a profit.* 9

ROBERT QUILLEN

## TAKE 1 MINUTE: for today's menu

### Breakfast

1 poached egg on wholegrain toast with a little butter, 1 kiwi fruit

### Lunch

chicken, apricot and almond salad
(*see* recipe page 160)

### Dinner

grilled trout with lemon and parsley,
4 grilled mushrooms, 2 tbsp leaf spinach,
2 tbsp mashed squash

10 black grapes

# 1 Three-limbed posture

This is an excellent forwards stretch for the back, releasing tension in the lumbar region. It also helps keep the hips, knees and feet flexible, massages the abdominal organs and is invaluable for promoting their health.

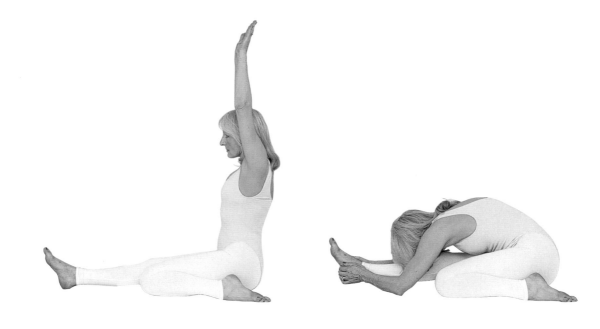

10 MINUTES IN THE MORNING

- Sit straight with both legs straight out in front of you. Place your left foot carefully by your left buttock.
- Inhale and stretch both arms in the air. Exhale and stretch forwards aiming to grab your right foot. Hold for 5, breathing normally. Then inhale, and return to an upright position. Exhale and relax.
- Repeat to the other side and then repeat the entire sequence twice.

### Extra Help
*It is really important to notice if one side is more flexible than the other. This can be due to many things, including imbalanced sports and poor posture. However, this movement will help you correct this potential problem. Sometimes, because of stiffness in the knees, ankles and feet, even placing your foot by your buttock can be very difficult in the beginning. Just practise doing this part of the movement, hold for a count of 5, and then try on the other side. Only when the foot is easily placed by the buttock should you continue with the movement.*

# 2 Pose of a sage

This movement tones the midriff and waistline, increases the flexibility and tone of the arms while releasing shoulder tension, stretches out the spine and tones the spinal nerves.

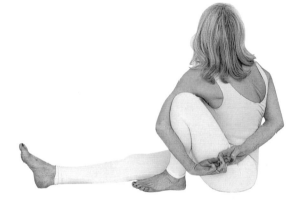

- Sit straight with both legs straight out in front of you. Place your left heel by your left buttock.
- Place your left arm straight out in front of you on the inside of your left knee and take your right arm back behind you and aim to join your hands together. If you can't join them, rest them where they are comfortable.
- Now correct your posture and sit very straight, inhale deeply and, as you exhale, rotate your upper body and turn your head over your right shoulder. Hold for a count of 5.
- Inhale and return your body forwards and face over your right leg. Exhale and gently bend forwards into your maximum position without strain. Your eventual aim is your chin to your right knee or shin. Hold your maximum forward stretch for a count of 5.
- Inhale as you return to an upright position. Exhale, relax and repeat to the other side, and then repeat the entire sequence once.

## Extra Help
*This movement can be very difficult in the beginning stages, first the hands won't join, second it is difficult to rotate the body keeping your spine straight, and third, even though you can do the backstretch, you find it difficult to place your chin on your knee in the forward stretch. It is the same for all of us – all I can say is that this movement reaches the bits that all other exercises leave out. Persevere and it will be well worth it! Do remember that you will benefit at every stage of this and every other movement.*

# 3   Pelvic tilt

A lovely movement to tone and tighten your bottom and tummy and release tension in your lower back.

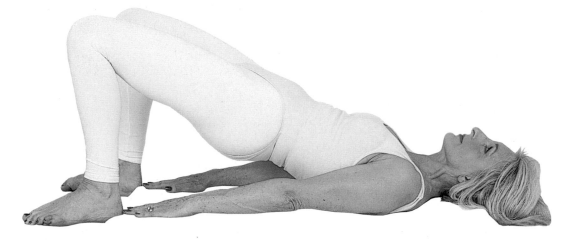

- Lie flat on your back. Place your feet about 1 foot apart and near your bottom, your fingertips just touching your heels.
- Inhale deeply and lift your bottom from the floor. In your maximum position exhale and really tighten your abdomen, pelvic floor and buttocks. Hold this position for a count of 5, breathing normally. Lower your bottom to the floor, relax and repeat 5 times.
- Draw your knees to your chest, interlock your hands around your knees, and gently rock your body from left to right 3 times, then gently let your legs stretch straight out in front of you and relax.

# TAKE 2 MINUTES: beauty tip

**Make it a great day –** Beauty honestly does come from the inside. We all have days when we feel downright low, depressed, fat and miserable but moods can be changed. Here are my favourite ways to convert a bad day into a great one.

1   Open the windows wide and look at the sky. Listen to the birds singing, look at the trees and flowers and enjoy.

2   Write down all the bad things you are thinking about yourself from your fat thighs to your spot on your chin, your dull hair to your untidy room. Write it all down and accept yourself just as you are. Now tear it up and put it in the bin.

3   Now write down your good points – *this is essential!* Do you have beautiful eyes, long legs, an infectious laugh? Write a list and paste this into your notebook.

4   Hug yourself. Tell yourself how lucky and loved you are.

5   Jump into the shower, wash and condition your hair.

6   Apply your best make-up and smile at yourself in the mirror.

7   Put on great clothes and smile again.

8   Have a good breakfast, fresh fruit, good organic yoghurt and a great cup of tea or coffee.

9   Read your blessings list.

10  Buy flowers for yourself. If on arrival at work you see someone else having a blue day, give them the flowers – it will make both of you feel better.

11  Remember, all of us feel inadequate at times. We feel we're not good enough, attractive enough, clever enough or kind enough. However, these feelings build fear inside each and everyone of us and this robs us of our ability to enjoy life and feel good about ourselves. So immediately look at your goals, count your blessings and remember this is not a rehearsal, this is *your* life. Decide to do your best with it – all of us are beautiful if we radiate a look of happiness and kindness and realize how lucky we are.

12  Make a list of places to visit or things you would like to do before your next milestone birthday. Would you like to ride on a husky driven sleigh in Greenland? Go whale watching? Scuba dive the Great Barrier Reef? Walk the Great Wall of China? Hike to Machu Picchu? Make your own list in your notebook and choose your priorities. Do something today to set the wheels in motion. Get excited, get moving, and have a wonderful day.

# DAY 25

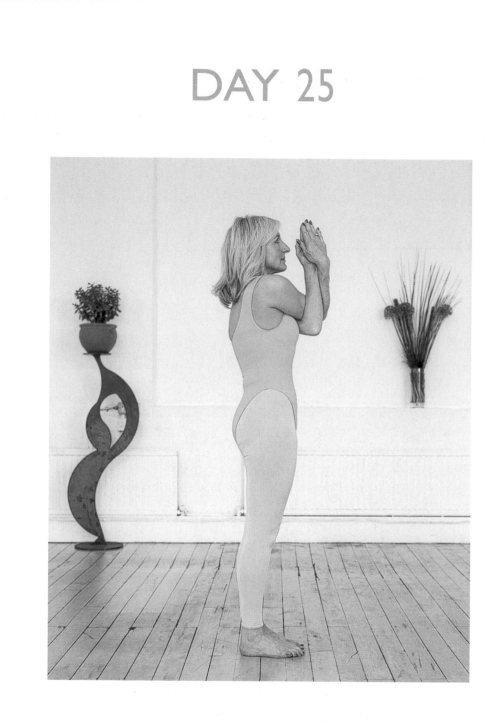

6 *Men often become what they believe themselves
to be. If I believe I cannot do something, it makes
me incapable of doing it. But when I believe I can,
then I acquire the ability to do it even if I didn't
have it in the beginning.* 9

MAHATMA GANDHI

## TAKE 2 MINUTES: to focus on your goals

Focus on your goals. Read them and do something to make them happen. At this stage you might feel slightly nervous about making yourself feel better and becoming thinner and more attractive. Maybe you feel it is nicer, easier and more comfortable to hide within a larger frame. Those thoughts are natural but really you do want your life to be better, to be slimmer, more attractive and more energetic. Challenge yourself to be the best you can – you can do it. You have got this far and in 3 more days you should be celebrating the fact that you are 10 lbs slimmer and feeling 10 times better.

Count your blessings and add at least 3 to your list.

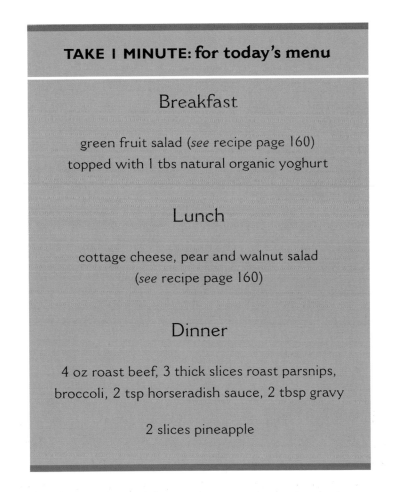

## TAKE 1 MINUTE: for today's menu

### Breakfast

green fruit salad (*see* recipe page 160)
topped with 1 tbs natural organic yoghurt

### Lunch

cottage cheese, pear and walnut salad
(*see* recipe page 160)

### Dinner

4 oz roast beef, 3 thick slices roast parsnips,
broccoli, 2 tsp horseradish sauce, 2 tbsp gravy

2 slices pineapple

# 1 Pose of a tortoise

This is an excellent movement for relieving stiffness in the lower back and hips. It tones the abdominal organs and the spine. It is a very soothing and refreshing movement.

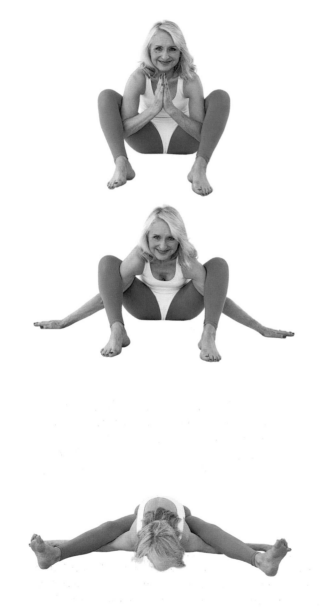

- Sit with your legs about 1 foot apart and your feet flat on the floor.
- Place your hands in prayer. Inhale and lower your elbows towards the floor. As you exhale, gently open your elbows and stretch your hands under your knees, placing them on the floor on the outer side of your knees.

- In your maximum stretch, notice the position of your elbows, if they are on the outer side of the knee you will be able to continue the movement. If not, just relax in your maximum position and hold for a count of 5, breathing normally.

- To continue the movement take another breath then stretch your legs out as wide as possible. As you stretch forwards, stretch your arms out as wide as possible.
- Relax in your maximum position without strain, aiming your chin to the floor and hold for a count of 10, breathing normally.
- Inhale and slowly and carefully draw in your feet, then your arms, and inhale as you return to the starting position. Exhale, relax and repeat once. Only when you can achieve the maximum stretch in tortoise with your chin on the floor and arms and legs at full stretch, you might like to try the advanced stage.
- For this, in your maximum tortoise stretch, gently take your arms behind your back and try to join your hands. Hold for 5, relax unclasp your hands, draw your feet in first and return slowly to your upright position, relax and repeat once.

# 2 Lowering your legs to the floor

**Caution:** If you have a weak lower back please read extra help first; do not do this movement if you are pregnant.

This movement is one of the best for helping you to that beautiful flat toned yoga tummy.

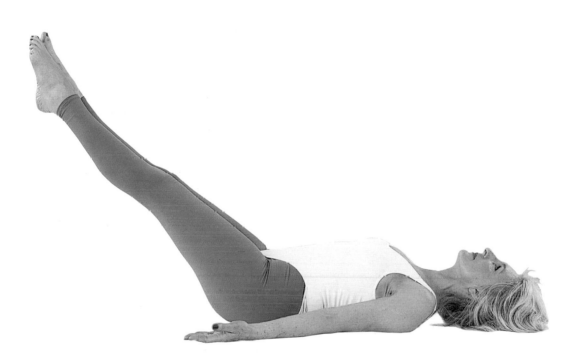

- Lie flat on your back with your arms by your sides.
- Bend your knees and gently lift your legs until they are at right angles to the floor.
- Inhale deeply and, as you exhale, carefully lower your legs all the way to the floor, keeping them straight. (In the beginning, it is best to lower your legs fairly quickly, slowing the movement down as your muscles become stronger.) Relax and repeat 3 times, increasing to 6 times as you progress in the movement.

## *Extra Help*
*When you do this movement to begin with, you may find that it is too strong for your lower back. If this is the case, lower your legs a little and when you feel the tiniest suggestion of a pull in the lower back, bend your knees and continue to lower your legs to the floor keeping your knees bent. Continue to practice like this and you will find that gradually you are able to lower your legs a little bit more until eventually you are able to lower them all the way to the floor without needing to bend them. You will then have considerably strengthened your lower back muscles and your abdominals.*

# 3   Shoulderstand

**Caution:** Do not attempt this movement if you have high blood pressure, any problems with your head and neck area, or if you are pregnant.

This movement is called the 'mother of yoga postures' and is the second most important yoga exercise – the first being the headstand. It has wonderful benefits, it stimulates excellent blood flow to the skin and hair and has a rejuvenating effect on them. It also helps to reverse the adverse aging effects of gravity. By stimulating extra blood flow to the thyroid and parathyroid glands in the neck it helps keep them in good condition and can help revitalize a sluggish metabolism.

The shoulderstand is also excellent for the health of the legs and can help prevent varicose veins, haemorrhoids and thread veins. It strengthens the spine, legs and abdominal muscles and the extra blood flow to the chest can be beneficial for asthma sufferers and the extra blood flow to the brain can help headache sufferers and benefit the brain itself, as well as improve eyesight and hearing.

* Lie flat on your back with your hands by your side. Take a deep breath in and, as you exhale, gently bend your knees and lift your lower body from the floor. Support your back
  by placing your hands at your waistline.
* Continue to lift your legs until your body is in a perfect straight line. This may take a while to achieve. Do your best without strain and then relax in your maximum movement.
* Hold your maximum position for a count of 10 to start with, increasing at the rate of about 30 seconds per week until you are holding for about 3 minutes.
* To come out of the posture, draw your knees to your forehead and then gently roll down your back about one vertebra at a time until your bottom touches the floor.
* Slide your hands under your buttocks and bring the top of your head on to the floor and relax in the position called 'pose of a fish'. Take a deep breath, hold for a count of 5, then exhale slowly and lower your upper body to the floor and lie flat. Close your eyes and relax.
* To finish, draw your knees to your chest and rock very gently from left to right to soothe your back and let it relax into the floor.
* Let both legs go straight out. Close your eyes and relax. Do not repeat.

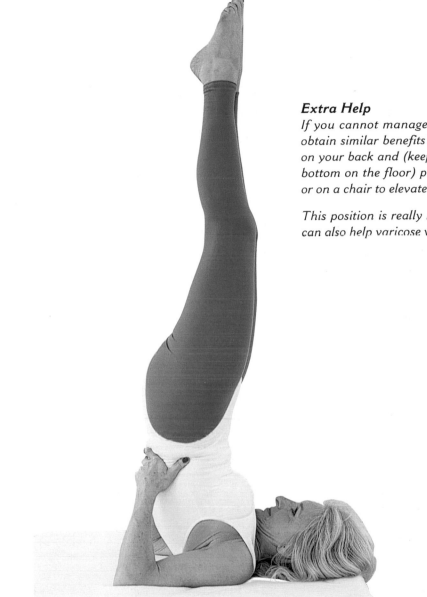

### Extra Help

*If you cannot manage this movement, you can obtain similar benefits for your legs by lying flat on your back and (keeping your upper body and bottom on the floor) placing your feet on a wall or on a chair to elevate them.*

*This position is really relaxing for tired legs and can also help varicose veins.*

## TAKE 2 MINUTES: lifestyle tip

**Create a 'good times book'** – This is a lovely thing to do and it is so much more than a photo album. Simply buy a pretty scrapbook and pile into it notes of your fabulous life moments. A happy dinner with friends, a great day on holiday, your daughter's first smile, the day you passed an exam. Don't make it too complicated, just make a small note of your great moments. This makes an uplifting read on blue days.

# DAY 26

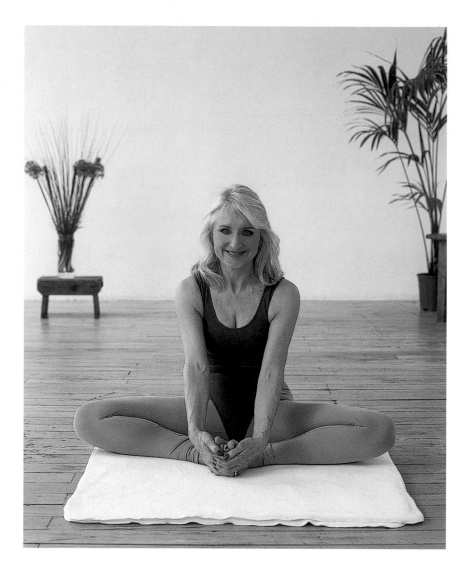

❝ *Twenty years from now you will be more disappointed by the things that you didn't do than by the ones you did do. So throw off the bowlines, sail away from the safe harbour, catch the trade winds in your sails. Explore, dream, discover.* ❞

MARK TWAIN

## TAKE 2 MINUTES: to focus on your goals

Continue to focus on your goals. I hope you now see the value of this daily focusing. It is also a great idea to make yourself a map or a scrapbook of your ideal life. Just as you have done with your daily visualization of your ideal body. Start collecting pictures of the lifestyle you would love. Include pictures of your ideal house, a map of where you would like to be; how you would like your garden to look; collect pictures of interiors you would love in your house. Include your ideal job and the amount of money you would like to earn each year Stick these pictures in a scrapbook or on a large cork board, remember the rules, daily focus and visualization will help them become a reality.

Count your blessings and be grateful for what you already have. Add 3 more to your list.

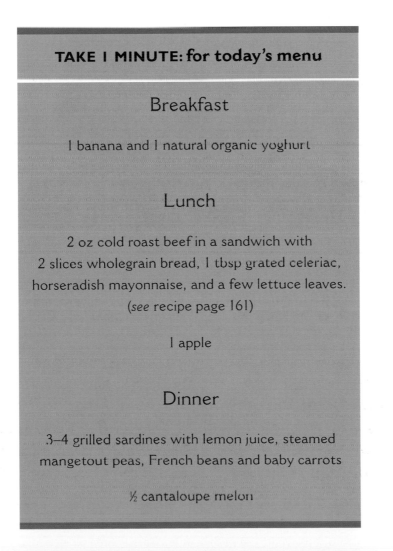

### TAKE 1 MINUTE: for today's menu

## Breakfast

1 banana and 1 natural organic yoghurt

## Lunch

2 oz cold roast beef in a sandwich with
2 slices wholegrain bread, 1 tbsp grated celeriac,
horseradish mayonnaise, and a few lettuce leaves.
(*see* recipe page 161)

1 apple

## Dinner

3–4 grilled sardines with lemon juice, steamed
mangetout peas, French beans and baby carrots

½ cantaloupe melon

# 1   Eye exercises

The eyes need exercises to keep them in good condition to strengthen the muscles, stimulate blood flow to the optic nerve and help prevent the lens stiffening. These movements do just that and can really help the eyesight. After practising these movements a lot of my pupils tell me that they no longer need their reading glasses. The exercises are most beneficial if you spend hour after hour on a computer.

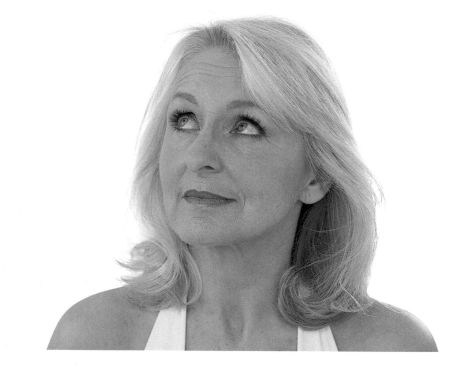

## EYE EXERCISE 1

- Sit straight and imagine an enormous clock in front of you. Look upward and your maximum upwards stretch is 12 o'clock. Hold for a count of 3 in this position, now move your eyes to 1 o'clock and again hold for a count of 3. Continue in this way round the clock until you once again arrive at 12 o'clock. Now go back the other way and continue round the clock until you once more reach 12 o'clock.

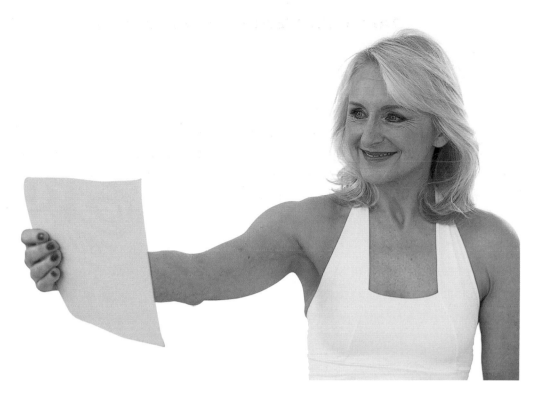

## EYE EXERCISE 2

* Find two pieces of print, one quite large that you are able to read easily without glasses or contact lenses and one that you have difficulty in reading but can just about manage in good light.
* Paste these pieces of print into your notebook.
* Look at them at least three times per day in excellent light: 1) at comfortable reading distance; 2) with your arm stretched out as far as possible; and 3) as near to your face you can before it goes blurry.
* Do this every day and you will find your eyesight benefiting. When this becomes easy for you then try two smaller pieces of print and continue. Once you have regained confidence in your ability to strengthen your eyesight, use this exercise with pieces of small print in your daily life, such as ingredient lists on bottles, and make it a lifetime habit. I am most grateful to have been taught these movements as at 62 years of age I still have no need for glasses. I find it very easy to fit these movements into the busiest day.
* After doing your eye exercises rub the palms of your hands together to warm them, then place your warmed hands over your closed eyes and stay in this position, breathing calmly and slowly for a count of 30. Then lower your hands, slowly open your eyes and relax. This is known as palming the eyes and is most refreshing for tired or strained eyes.

Now you have worked your eye muscles it is a wonderful thing to relax in the pose of a plough (*see* page 98). This will stimulate blood flow to your face, scalp, brain and eyes and release tension in your lower back.

# 2 Deep relaxation

This is the most difficult thing to teach the average pupil who feels that she is too busy to relax. This feeling of non-stop action and pressure can lead to chronic tension which inhibits the flow of blood and lymph to our tissues. This can lead to weakness and eventually disease can result. Yoga exercises systematically go through the entire body carefully stretching out the tension within. And this, along with the slow deep breathing in every position, results in a lovely feeling of calm and peace.

When the tension is removed it is much easier to relax both body and mind. This results in increased flow of blood to all the tissues, benefiting each and every cell, and the lymphatic system resumes its normal function removing toxins and fighting infection in our bodies. Blood pressure, which rises under tension slowly returns to normal.

When the mind relaxes, it becomes calm and peaceful, clarity is restored, muddled thinking vanishes, problems seem easier to solve and new creative ideas arrive out of the blue. As you continue to practise relaxation you will discover the happiness and peace within you. All this has a huge effect on your appearance, skin and hair. Nothing is more aging than tension and nothing is worse for your skin and hair.

As you learn to relax your mind and body, your skin will regain its radiant glow, and your hair its bounce and shine due to the circulation being restored in this area. And once you realize that happiness is inside you and yours for the taking, the lines of tension will gradually fade away resulting in a youthful radiance and passion and new energy for living.

Practise this whenever you feel tired or tense. It works wonders!

*"Beauty without self-confidence is less attractive than ugliness with self-confidence. If you are confident you are beautiful."*

GEORGE CUKOR

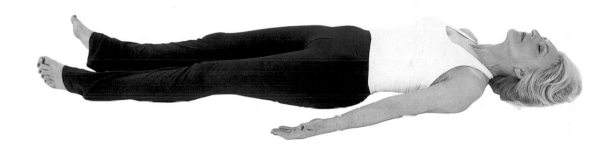

- Lie flat on your back on your mat, your feet about 2 ft apart and your arms palms uppermost about 1 ft from your body.
- Make sure that you are warm enough. In colder weather it is wise to cover yourself with a blanket as your temperature may drop as your body relaxes.
- Slow your breathing down, breathing calmly, slowly and deeply inhaling and exhaling through your nose.
- Relax your feet, ankles, and calves. Relax your thighs now feel your legs becoming heavy and really relaxed.
- Relax your abdomen and your back. Relax your chest and shoulders.
- Relax your arms and feel them becoming heavy, sinking on to the floor.

- Smooth out your facial muscles, keeping your breathing slow and deep. Let your eyelids become heavy and roll your eyeballs upwards. Let your scalp slide back and let your body relax into a calm and dreamy, drowsy state.
- With your body relaxed, visualize beautiful snow-covered mountains sparkling in the sunlight. Keep this in your mind and relax, relax, relax.
- Stay there relaxing for 5–10 minutes.
- Slowly dismiss your picture, take a deep breath, stretch your entire body, then grab your right knee and gently pull yourself up into a sitting position.

# TAKE 2 MINUTES: lifestyle tip

## Learn to meditate

Living in today's high-pressure world can be full of stress, anxiety and tension. We resort to the usual remedies – such as coffee, alcohol and sleeping pills – but these only work on the symptoms, not the cause. Over 5,000 years ago, the yogis of ancient India realized that by learning to quieten the mind by meditating we can help ourselves to a feeling of calm and peace and, in doing so, alleviate the damaging effects of stress.

When the mind is thinking hard it is busy and frequently overloaded with worries about the past and anxieties about the future, the brain in this state emits rapid beta brain waves. Once you start to calm the mind and focus on one object or your breathing, the mind stays in the present, free from stressful thoughts. When this feeling of calm and peace flows through your being, your brain will start to emit slower, more rhythmic alpha brain waves. This lovely peaceful sense of calm pervades our whole being, breathing slows down and stress hormone levels and blood pressure fall. Meditators find that they are less prone to stress and depression, they have more energy, need less sleep and look younger and more radiant then non-meditators.

There are many meditation techniques and you will need to find the method that works best for you. To get you started, the following technique is my preferred method of meditation.

Early morning is traditionally a good time for meditation but if your house is in chaos then choose a time when you can relax and enjoy the peace and calm.

Sit in a comfortable position with your back straight, the lotus position is ideal but by no means essential; if you are not yet comfortable in it then a crossed-leg position, kneeling position or your favourite armchair will do fine.

Make sure that you are warm enough as your temperature can drop a little during meditation.

Make sure that you will not be disturbed. If you have an appointment later, it is a good idea to set your alarm clock for the end of your allocated meditation time – it is not unusual to fall asleep during your first meditation sessions.

Close your eyes and concentrate on your breathing. Don't try to change it or regulate it, just bring your attention to it.

If your mind wanders, and it does for the most experienced meditator, bring your attention back to your breathing. Don't think that you are bad at meditating if your mind wanders, just relax and gently bring your mind back to your breathing and allow all other thoughts to just slip away.

Start with 10 minutes of meditation and gradually increase it to 20 minutes.

Don't expect instant results, meditation does require practice. You will benefit from all your meditations and eventually you will feel clear, calm and focused. Frequently you will receive new insights into a particular area of your life and problems will seem easier to solve. Once you have been meditating for a while you will realize that you manifest your own destiny, and experience a beautiful inner joy and confidence, and nothing is impossible for you.

Other ways of meditating include focusing on a special object like a beautiful flower, a piece of crystal or rock, a candle flame (make sure that it is safe if you are liable to fall asleep) or a religious symbol (in fact, any single object that works for you is fine). Some people prefer to repeat a mantra. Choose a word like 'peace' or 'calm' or the yoga word *om* (pronounced *aum*), meaning 'what was, what is and what shall be'. Take a deep breath in and as you exhale say it softly and slowly making your exhalation and the sound last as long as possible, then repeat it over and over again until a feeling of peace flows through you.

# DAY 27

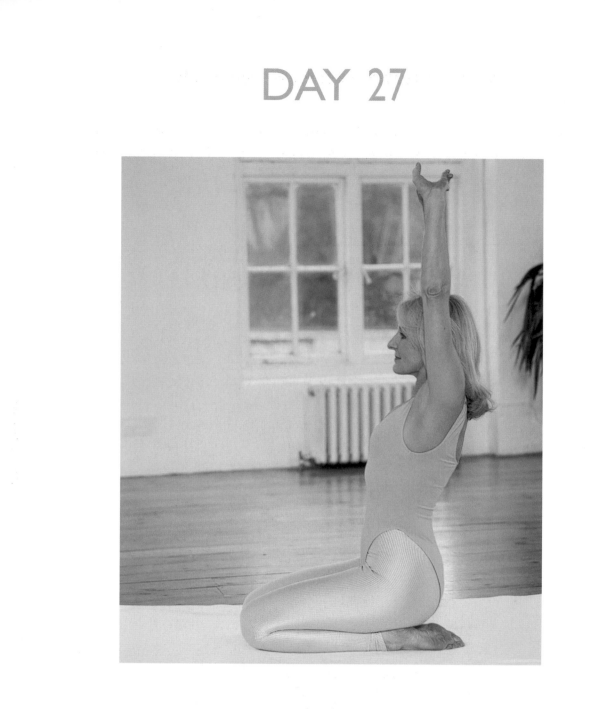

❝ For a long time it had seemed to me that life was about to begin – real life. But there was always some obstacle in the way, something to be got through first, some unfinished business, time still to be saved, a debt to be paid. Then life would begin. At last it dawned on me that these obstacles were my life. ❞

ALFRED D'SOUZA

# TAKE 2 MINUTES: to focus on your goals

Focus on your goals and visualize them. Take a minute to count your blessings and add at least 3 more to your ever-growing list. Don't put off happiness until you have accomplished your goals. Just *be happy today*.

## TAKE I MINUTE: for today's menu

### Breakfast

½ papaya filled with blueberries, topped with
1 tbsp natural organic yoghurt.

### Lunch

Bacon, lettuce and tomato sandwich
(*see* recipe page 161)

2 kiwi fruit

### Dinner

4 oz grilled tuna on a bed of cooked spinach;
tomato, onion and salad with 2 tsp balsamic
vinegar and olive oil dressing

3 fresh dates

# TAKE 25 MINUTES: for today's exercises

It is time to do your 27th day yoga workout, using all the exercises you have learned this week. It will take you about 25 minutes.

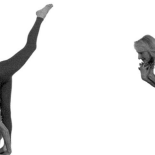

• The triangle

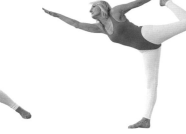

• Dancer's posture

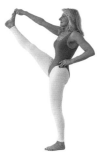

• Big toe balance

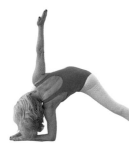

• Head to knee balance

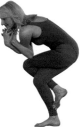

• Eagle balance

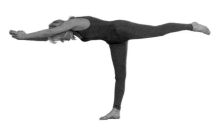

• Standing stick balance

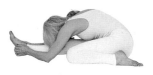

• Three-limbed posture

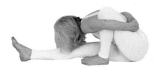

• Pose of a sage

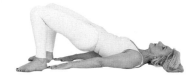

• Pelvic tilt

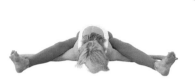

- Pose of a tortoise

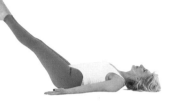

- Lowering your legs to the floor

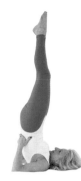

- Shoulderstand

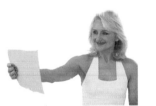

- Eye exercises

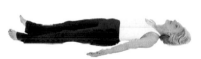

- Deep relaxation

## TAKE 2 MINUTES: lifestyle tip

**Remove your energy drainers.** There are many things in life that act as a drain on our natural energy flow. These can come in many shapes or forms, such as an untidy desk, dead flowers, insufficient fresh air, negative people, a pile of unanswered mail, too much clutter, a broken food blender, etc. It is a good idea to go through your top energy drainers, write them down, put in your diary a time to fix them and how you will attend to them and try over the next few weeks to complete your top 6 items. You will be amazed at the energy release it will give you.

# DAY 28

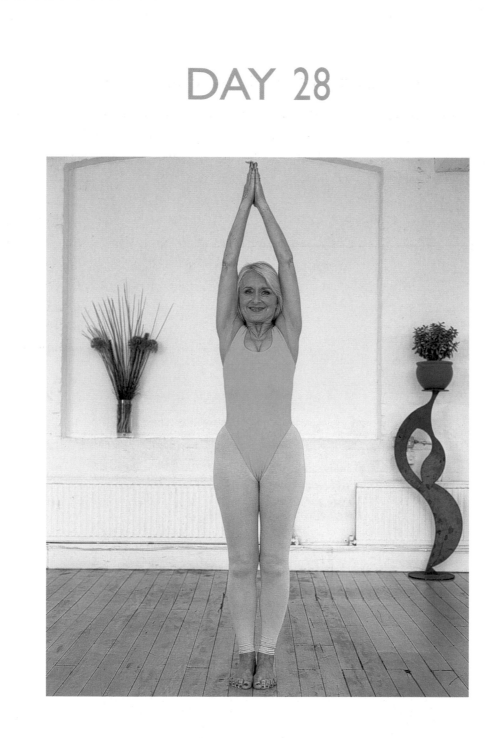

❛ The future belongs to those who believe
in the beauty of their dreams. ❜

ELEANOR ROOSEVELT

## TAKE 2 MINUTES: to focus on your goals

Well done, you have made it! Now it's time to fill in your new measurements and weight in your notebook. I do hope you are feeling fantastic and you have enjoyed this 28-day plan. We have covered a lot of topics and you have learnt many new exercises. I really hope you feel and look better than you have for ages.

**Lotus Flower Legend** – Picture a dark muddy pond and in the mud see a tiny seed. Watch the seed grow a root and shoot and watch the journey of the shoot to the surface of the pond. On the way, it will encounter reeds, debris, frogs, fish but it keeps focusing on the light shining on the top of the pond. Eventually it reaches the top and opens into a beautiful lotus flower. If we learn from the lotus flower, focus daily on our goals and treat the problems and obstacles each day as necessary stepping stones on life's incredible journey, something very beautiful will be the result. So keep visualizing your goals and meanwhile enjoy each day.

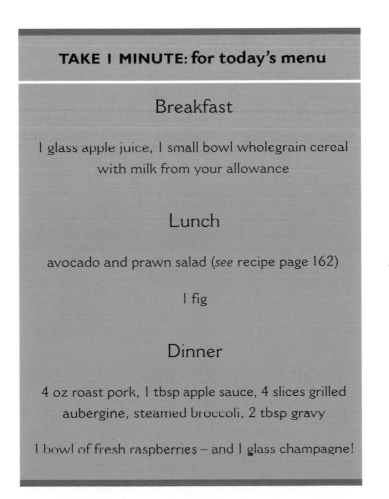

## TAKE 1 MINUTE: for today's menu

### Breakfast

1 glass apple juice, 1 small bowl wholegrain cereal with milk from your allowance

### Lunch

avocado and prawn salad (*see* recipe page 162)

1 fig

### Dinner

4 oz roast pork, 1 tbsp apple sauce, 4 slices grilled aubergine, steamed broccoli, 2 tbsp gravy

1 bowl of fresh raspberries – and 1 glass champagne!

## TAKE 25 MINUTES: for today's exercises

Today, go for a wonderful long walk.

---

### TAKE 2 MINUTES: lifestyle tip

Keep dreaming, keep setting goals, never give up, keep doing new things; live, love and laugh and this will keep the twinkle in your eye and keep you young and beautiful forever.

---

# And finally …

If 10 lbs was all you had to lose – but if you have enjoyed eating this way and doing the exercises, then just slowly increase the portion sizes but stick to the basic plan. If your weight goes up again, then simply cut back to the basic plan. You will soon be able to adjust the plan so you can keep slim and healthy for life.

If you still have weight to lose, simply continue with the plan until you have lost all your excess weight and then adjust it as mentioned above. Remember, keep your goals in mind and do let me know how you progress. You can write to me c/o my publishers.

Wishing you a very healthy, happy, slim and exciting future.

With my love

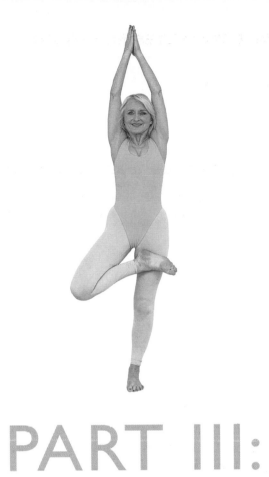

# PART III:

# THE RECIPES

# Salads and Sandwiches

## Salad Niçoise (serves 1)

mixed fresh salad leaves
10 cooked French beans
6 black olives
3½ oz tuna fish and 3 anchovies
2 sliced tomatoes
6 slices cucumber
1 tbsp vinaigrette (*see* recipe page 170)
1 clove garlic

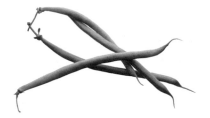

Rub the salad bowl with garlic. Fill with the salad leaves. Add the French beans, olives, tomatoes and cucumber. Place the tuna on top in bite-sized pieces. Just before serving, sprinkle with a little parsley and toss with the vinaigrette dressing

## Chicken and papaya salad (serves 2)

2 cooked chicken breasts (skinned)
1 tbsp parsley
1 tbsp mayonnaise (*see* recipe page 169)
1 ripe papaya
mixed salad leaves

Take the chicken breasts and cut into cubes. Peel the papaya and cut it into quarters, remove all the seeds. Cut ¾ of the papaya into neat bite-size chunks and mix with the chicken. Mash the remaining papaya and mix with the mayonnaise. Gently mix the chicken and papaya with the mayonnaise until it is evenly coated. Pile on top of the salad leaves, sprinkle with chopped parsley and serve immediately. (This looks and tastes so good people will ask you for the recipe!)

# Avocado, spinach and bacon salad (serves 1)

½ avocado, cubed
6 black olives
2 tomatoes, sliced
6 slices cucumber
fresh spinach
1 tbsp vinaigrette dressing
3 rashers grilled bacon (hot if possible)
1 clove garlic

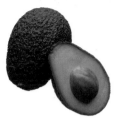

Crush the garlic and place in the bowl with the spinach. Add all the other salad ingredients and toss in the salad dressing and top with the bacon (cut into ½ inch pieces) and serve immediately. Delicious!

# Endive, walnut and blue cheese salad (serves 1)

1 or 2 endives
1½ oz blue cheese
black pepper
6 chopped walnuts
parsley
1 tbsp caesar salad dressing (*see* recipe page 155)

Arrange the endive leaves on a plate. Top with the walnuts and crumble the blue cheese and place on top. Drizzle the dressing over the top. (I use this recipe as a delicious light lunch or it is great as a starter for a dinner party.)

# Tomato, basil and onion salad (serves 2)

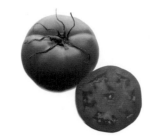

4 large tomatoes thinly sliced

1 tbsp chopped basil

1 red onion sliced

1 clove finely chopped garlic

1 tbsp olive oil

1 lemon

salt and pepper to taste

Place the tomatoes in a bowl. Cover with the onion and basil. Mix the garlic, salt, pepper, olive oil and lemon juice together and pour over the tomatoes.

# Prawn salad (serves 1)

4 oz cooked prawns

4 black olives

2 sliced tomatoes

1 sliced red onion

mixed salad leaves

2 tsp marie rose dressing (*see* recipe page 169)

2 tsp vinaigrette

pinch of paprika

Place all the salad ingredients in the bowl and toss in the vinaigrette dressing. Gently coat the prawns in the marie rose dressing and place on top. Sprinkle with paprika. (Again, this is an easy starter for a dinner party and very popular!)

# Greek salad (serves 1)

2 oz feta cheese

¼ cucumber

3 tomatoes

8 black olives

½ green pepper

1 red onion

3 sprigs oregano

1 tbsp olive oil and balsamic vinegar dressing

Halve the cucumber and remove the seeds. Peel and chop it into ½in cubes and place in a bowl. Quarter the tomatoes and cut into wedges, add the black olives. Finely slice the onion and pepper and add to the cucumber and tomato. Sprinkle over the oregano and, just before serving, toss in the oil and vinegar dressing and add the cheese place on a bed of salad leaves and season to taste.

## Caesar salad (serves 2)

1 large cos lettuce, washed and torn into bite-sized pieces
4 oz grated parmesan cheese
4 fillets anchovy
2 tbsp Caesar salad dressing (*see* recipe page 170)

Place the torn lettuce and parmesan in a bowl and toss in the Caesar dressing. Top with the anchovies.

## Chicken and mango salad (serves 2)

2 cooked chicken breasts (skinned)
1 ripe fresh mango
2 tbsp fresh mayonnaise
1 cos lettuce
2 tomatoes neatly sliced
6 black olives
mixed salad sprouts

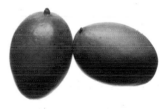

Peel the mango and cut into neat slices. Take ¼ of mango and mash it with the mayonnaise. Wash the lettuce leaves, drain and arrange on a pretty circular plate, add the tomatoes, olives and a few slices of mango in a circular arrangement. Cut the chicken into bite-sized cubes and chop the remaining mango into small pieces. Toss in the mayonnaise until it is evenly coated and place on the salad leaves. Top with the sprouts and serve immediately.

# Carrot and apple salad (serves 2)

**4 large carrots**
**1 red apples**
**1 tbsp chopped chives**
**1 tbsp mayonnaise**

Coarsely grate the carrots and apple and mix with the chives and mayonnaise. This is delicious!

# Mozzarella, tomato and basil salad (serves 1)

**2 oz buffalo mozzarella**
**4 tomatoes – large, red and ripe**
**6 sprigs of basil**
**8 cos lettuce leaves**
**1 tbsp olive oil**
**a few drops balsamic vinegar**
**salt and freshly ground black pepper**

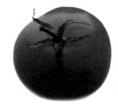

On a large plate arrange first the lettuce leaves, then the slices of tomatoes alternating with thin slices of mozzarella. Place a leave of basil between each slice. Sprinkle the cracked black pepper and a little sea salt to taste over the salad and finally drizzle over the olive oil and balsamic vinegar. Serve immediately.

# Smoked salmon, asparagus and lettuce sandwich

**2 oz smoked salmon**
**shredded lettuce**
**6 asparagus spears (cooked)**
**2 slices wholegrain bread**
**a little butter or mayonnaise**
**squeeze of lemon**

Butter bread lightly and cover 1 slice with shredded lettuce. Place the smoked salmon on top and finally the asparagus. Sprinkle with sea salt and freshly ground black pepper to taste and a small squeeze of lemon. Top with the other slice of bread and enjoy.

# Grilled goat's cheese on mixed leaf salad (serves 1)

mixed salad leaves
a few mixed sprouts
2 oz goat's cheese
2 small thin slices of a wholegrain baguette
2 tsp olive oil
a few drops balsamic vinegar
1 tbsp chopped mixed herbs (parsley, thyme, coriander, chives, basil)

Toss the salad in the olive oil with the herbs, add vinegar to taste and place on a plate. Lightly toast the thin slices of baguette, then place the goat's cheese on top of them. Place under the grill at least 8 in from the heat source and grill until the top of the cheese is just turning brown and the rest is heated through. Place on top of the salad, sprinkle with the bean sprouts and serve immediately.

# Mixed seafood salad (serves 1)

oil and vinegar dressing
4 oz mixed cooked seafood (such as, mussels, cockles, prawns, squid – most supermarkets now sell an excellent mix of cooked seafood)
few drops balsamic vinegar
1 tbsp olive oil
½ lettuce
8 leaves fresh basil
½ clove fresh garlic
10 leaves of parsley
1 onion
2 tomatoes
½ lemon
salt and freshly ground black pepper

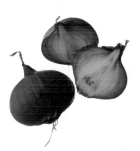

Chop the herbs and crush the garlic. Put in a bowl. Peel the onion, finely chop and add to this mixture. Chop the tomatoes and also place in the bowl, now add the seafood. Mix in a separate bowl the oil and vinegar and a little of the lemon juice with salt and pepper to taste. Add to the seafood mix and toss carefully. Arrange the lettuce on a plate, add the seafood and serve immediately.

# Smoked trout with cucumber, pine nuts and pepper salad (serves 2)

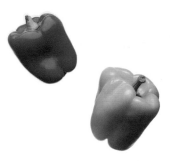

2 smoked trout
1 lemon cut into wedges
1 red pepper and 1 yellow pepper
½ cucumber
10 leaves coriander
1 tbsp mayonnaise
1 tsp horseradish sauce
1 tbsp pine nuts
a handful rocket

Remove the seeds from the pepper and chop into small pieces. Peel and chop the cucumber, chop the coriander and mix with the pepper and pine nuts in a bowl. Combine the mayonnaise with the horseradish and add to the cucumber mixture. Serve the smoked trout on a few leaves of rocket, garnished with the lemon wedges, with the cucumber mix on the side.

# Fresh crab and mango salad (serves 2)

1 mango
8 oz white crab meat
1 cos lettuce
1 bunch watercress
10 black olives
4 tomatoes
a few sprouts
1 tbsp mayonnaise
1 tbsp olive oil
juice of 1 lemon
salt and freshly ground black pepper

Peel the mango and cut into neat slices and set aside. Mash ¼ of the mango and mix with the mayonnaise. Arrange the lettuce on 2 plates with the wide part of the leaf at the outside of the plate and narrow part in the middle. Place the watercress on top of the lettuce, then the tomatoes and olives. Place the crab in the middle of the plate and top with the mango mayonnaise mix. Decorate with the mango slices and top with the sprouts. Whisk the oil, lemon and pepper and salt together and drizzle a little over the salad. Serve immediately. Crab and mango go especially well together and this pretty dish is ideal for a light lunch or a dinner party starter.

## Red coleslaw (serves 4)

½ red cabbage (shredded)
½ white cabbage (shredded)
1 red apple grated
1 tbsp raisins
salt and freshly ground black pepper
1 tbsp good mayonnaise mixed with 1 tbsp organic natural yoghurt.

Mix all the ingredients together and serve immediately.

## Chicken Waldorf salad (serves 2)

2 chicken breasts (cooked)
1 green apple
8 chopped walnut halves
½ fresh lemon
2 sticks celery
1 lettuce
salt and pepper
1 tbsp natural organic yoghurt
1 tbsp mayonnaise
1 cos lettuce

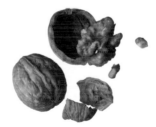

Cut the apple into small chunks, squeeze the lemon juice over them, then place in a bowl. Cut the celery into similar size chunks and add to the apple. Add most of the walnuts. Cut the chicken into small bite-size pieces and add the celery, apple and walnut. Mix the mayonnaise with the yoghurt and add to the chicken mixture, carefully coating the chicken, apples and celery. Wash and dry the lettuce and arrange on a large plate. Place the chicken mixture on top and garnish with the remaining walnuts.

# Chicken, apricot and almond salad (serves 2)

8 oz diced cooked chicken
6 diced ripe apricots
10 almonds, thinly sliced or chopped
1 tbsp mayonnaise
1 tbsp natural yoghurt
2 teaspoons apricot or mango chutney
mixed green salad leaves and watercress

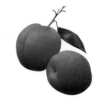

Place the chicken and all but 1 tbsp apricots and the almonds into a bowl. Mix the mayonnaise, yoghurt and apricot chutney together and add to the chicken mixture. Arrange the salad leaves on 2 plates and divide the mixture equally and place in the centre of each plate. Surround with the watercress and garnish with the saved apricots.

# Green fruit salad (serves 1)

1 apple
1 kiwi fruit
1 slice honeydew melon
6 grapes
1 tsp runny honey
1 sprig mint

Slice all the fruits into attractive slices and put in a bowl. Warm the honey and drizzle it over the top. Garnish with a sprig of mint. (This is delicious and refreshing, ideal on a summer's day as a light refreshing dessert.)

# Cottage cheese, pear and walnut salad (serves 2)

12 oz cottage cheese
1 sliced ripe pear
10 chopped walnut halves
rocket, lettuce, watercress and salad sprouts
1 tbsp dressing olive oil and balsamic vinegar dressing

Wash and dry the salad leaves. Place them in a bowl and toss in the dressing, then arrange on a large plate. Place the cottage cheese in the middle and surround with the sliced fresh pear. Sprinkle the chopped walnuts and salad sprouts over the leaves and serve immediately.

# Roast beef sandwich with celeriac grated with horseradish mayonnaise (serves 1)

2 oz roast beef
2 slices wholegrain bread, lightly buttered
salad greens
a few salad sprouts
2 tbsp grated celeriac mixed with 2 tsp mayonnaise mixed
   with 1 tsp horseradish sauce

Mix the celeriac with the mayonnaise and horseradish and spread half of it over a slice of wholegrain bread. Place one slice of beef on top, then the lettuce, then the other slice of roast beef and finally the rest of the celeriac mixture and the other slice of bread.

# Bacon, lettuce and tomato sandwich (serves 1)

2 oz grilled bacon
shredded lettuce
1 sliced tomato
2 slices wholegrain bread, lightly buttered

Place the bacon directly on the first slice of bread. Cover with the lettuce and tomato, place the other slice of bread on top and serve immediately.

# Tomato and onion salad (serves 1)

2 ripe plum tomatoes
1 small red onion
a few chopped chives
2 tsp olive oil
a few drops balsamic vinegar
salt and pepper to taste

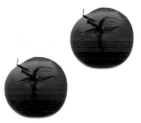

Thinly slice the tomatoes and onion. Place in a dish and season to taste. Sprinkle the chives over the top and drizzle over the olive oil and finally the balsamic vinegar.

# Avocado and prawn salad (serves 1)

½ avocado

salad leaves – endive, lettuce, watercress

2 tomatoes quartered

6 slices cucumber

6 black olives

2 oz prawns

2 tsp marie rose dressing (*see* recipe page 169)

2 tsp olive oil

a few drops balsamic vinegar

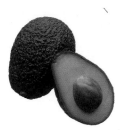

Wash and dry the salad leaves and place in a bowl. Add the tomatoes, cucumber and black olives. Carefully toss in the olive oil and balsamic vinegar. Peel and dice the avocado and place on top of the salad leaves, then add the prawns in the centre. Cover the prawns in the marie rose sauce.

# Green salad with olive oil and lemon (serves 1)

mixed salad greens, washed and dried

chopped fresh herbs

1 clove garlic

1 tbsp olive oil

juice of ½ lemon

salt and freshly ground black pepper

Rub the clove of garlic around a salad bowl and then add the salad greens. Add the oil and toss until all the leaves are coated in the oil. Add the lemon juice and toss again. Season with salt and freshly ground black pepper adding chopped fresh herbs according to taste.

# Fish

## Grilled salmon with pesto, mashed squash & steamed broccoli (serves 2)

2 × 6 oz salmon steaks
4 tbsp pesto (*see* page 170)
1 tbsp olive oil
lemon juice

Place the salmon steaks on the grill. Drizzle olive oil over them and squeeze on the lemon juice. Grill until done. Remove from the grill and spread with the pesto. Return to the grill for about 2 minutes or until the pesto just starts to brown. Serve immediately with the squash and the broccoli.

## Roast sea bass with lemon & parsley butter with wild mushrooms & steamed French beans (serves 2)

1 large or 2 small sea bass
16 cleaned wild mushrooms
juice of 1 lemon
1 fresh lemon
2 tbsp unsalted butter
1 tbsp fresh chopped parsley
2 cloves crushed garlic
salt and freshly ground black pepper

Ask your fishmonger to clean and scale your sea bass for you. Make 5 cuts on each side of the fish. Mix 1 tbsp butter, 2 cloves crushed garlic, fresh chopped parsley and the juice of one lemon and push into the cuts. Melt the rest of the butter, mix and toss in the mushrooms. Put the fish into a roasting pan on buttered silver foil surrounded by the mushrooms and roast at 200°C for about 20 minutes or until well done (depending on size and thickness of your fish). Serve with the remaining lemon cut into quarters. Season to taste with the sea salt and freshly ground black pepper.

# Sole Veronique

2 × 6 oz sole fillets
a little butter
½ pint fish stock
1 glass white wine or dry vermouth
20 seedless green grapes
1 lemon
salt and freshly ground black pepper
4 tbsp double cream

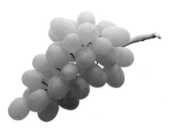

Grill the sole in an ovenproof dish. Once ready cover with foil and keep warm. To make the sauce: place the juices from the sole, the fish stock, wine or vermouth in a saucepan and reduce to about 1 small cupful or less (a syrupy texture is needed). Add the grapes to the sauce and cook again for about 2–3 minutes, being careful not to squash them. Add a squeeze of lemon juice, finally carefully add the cream and slowly simmer a little to get that beautiful creamy consistency (make sure it doesn't boil). Season to taste and serve. This is great for a dinner party.

# Scallops with ginger and grapefruit (serves 2)

2 tbsp soy sauce
1 grapefruit, peeled and segmented
1 tbsp olive oil
2 tbsp grated fresh ginger
1 tsp mustard
2 tsp honey
½ lb fresh scallops or 8 big ones or 10 small ones

Stir together the honey, ginger, soy sauce and mustard and set aside. In a frying pan heat the oil, add the scallops and seal quickly. Turn the heat down and add the soy sauce mixture. Mix and toss the scallops in this sauce. Just before they are done, toss the grapefruit segments in the frying pan until golden brown and serve with the scallops and celeriac. Serve with a side dish of freshly cooked spinach.

# Moules marinière

2 lbs mussels
1 oz butter
3 onions finely chopped
1 clove garlic finely chopped
2 glasses white wine
1 tbsp parsley, finely chopped

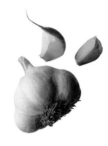

Clean the mussels and remove barnacles and fibrous 'beards', discard any that are open. Put the mussels, onion, garlic and butter into a large pan and add the wine. Bring to the boil, cover the pan and cook over a high heat for about 5 mins, shaking the pan occasionally. Place the mussels into a large bowl discarding any that have remained closed and keep warm. Reduce the liquid until it is a nice soup-like consistency. Add ½ the parsley to the liquid and pour over the mussels. Sprinkle with the remaining parsley and serve immediately.

# Meat and Poultry

## Pork steaks with red apples, spinach & swede (serves 2)

2 pork steaks, 4–5 oz each

2 red apples

1 tbsp olive oil

1 tbsp balsamic vinegar

1 tbsp sage

leaf spinach

1 whole swede

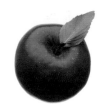

Place the pork steaks in a dish with the oil, vinegar and sage spooned over them. Slice the apples into large circles and remove the core. Heat the butter in a large frying pan and drop in the apples and cook for 3–4 mins or until they are golden brown. Keep them warm. Remove the pork from the marinade and cook in the frying pan for about 5 mins on each side or until completely cooked. Top with the apple and serve with steamed leaf spinach and mashed swede.

## Chicken and bacon with tomato sauce (serves 2)

2 chicken breasts

2 rashers bacon

2 onions

1 clove garlic

1 tbsp olive oil

salt and freshly ground black pepper

1 small jar organic tomato and basil sauce

2 tsp chopped fresh parsley, thyme and basil mix

Heat a little of the oil in a large frying pan, add the finely sliced onion and the chopped garlic and gently fry. Remove the rind from the bacon and cut into strips, add them to the onion, mix and gently sauté. Now add the rest of the olive oil and the chicken breasts and gently cook for a few minutes turning the chicken until it is sealed and starts to brown on all sides. Now add the tomato and basil sauce, cover the pan and cook slowly until the chicken is thoroughly cooked (about 20 mins). This is delicious – serve with French beans.

# Beef hotpot (serves 2)

This is a lovely heart-warming winter dish. I normally prepare it after a light lunch on Sunday, pop it in the oven and slow cook, enjoying at dinner after a long walk in the country.

3 large carrots peeled and cut into thick slices
3 large onions peeled and cut into thick slices
1 clove garlic
10 oz braising beef cut into cubes
1 glass good red wine
1 tbsp olive oil
salt and pepper
1 organic stock cube
½ pint water
1 tbsp fresh or dried thyme
2 tsp parsley and a little sage

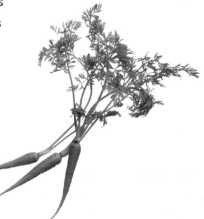

Place the oil in a large saucepan and heat it until hot. Add the onions and garlic, let them cook a little and then add the beef and carrots. Seal the beef all over; then add the wine, water, stock cubes and herbs. Gently bring to the boil, then simmer gently for about 5 minutes. Cover and place in the oven at 150–170°C for about 5 hours, or place in a slow cooker if you have one. Before serving, place the beef and vegetables in a dish and keep warm. Reduce the liquid until it is a lovely rich gravy, return to the meat and vegetables and serve with celeriac mash.

If you prefer a thicker gravy, then mix a small knob of butter in a bowl with 2 tsp wholegrain organic flour, add 2 tbsp of the gravy to this, mix it in, and then carefully add to the rest of the sauce. Bring to the boil and then cook for 2–3 mins before returning the sauce to the beef and vegetables.

# Vegetable Dishes

## Celeriac in mustard mayonnaise (serves 2)

1 whole celeriac
2 tbs mayonaise
2 tsp wholegrain mustard

Grate the celeriac and mix with the mayonnaise and wholegrain mustard.

## Ratatouille (serves 4)

2 tbsp good olive oil
2 onions
1 aubergine
2 red peppers
2 courgettes
8 chopped fresh tomatoes
4 tbsp tomato puree or organic tomato and basil sauce
4 cloves garlic
1 bunch mixed herbs

In a large saucepan, heat the oil and gently sauté the onions and garlic, add the aubergine, courgettes and pepper and sauté for a further 5 mins. Add the tomatoes and herbs and continue to sauté these vegetables. Finally, add the tomato puree, stir and leave to simmer for about 30 mins, finally add salt and pepper to taste. This is a delicious fresh vegetable dish. There are many variations but this is my favourite.

## Mashed parsnips (serves 2)

4 large parsnips
1 tsp butter
salt and pepper

Peel and cut the parsnips into large slices. Steam or boil until soft. Mash into a creamy consistency and add the butter, salt and pepper.

# Sauces and Dressings

## Tomato salsa

2 large ripe tomatoes

2 tbsp organic tomato ketchup

2 tsp cider vinegar

1 tbsp olive oil

a few drops Worcestershire sauce

½ tsp French mustard

Salt and freshly ground black pepper

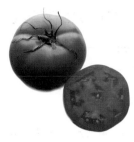

Chop the tomatoes coarsely and mix with the remainder of the ingredients. Season to taste and serve.

## Mayonnaise

3 egg yolks

1 tbsp warm water

1 tsp fresh mustard

1 tbsp wine vinegar, cider vinegar or lemon juice

1 pint very light olive oil

salt and freshly ground black pepper

Place the egg yolks, warm water and mustard in your blender and blend for a few seconds. Pour the oil slowly through the funnel as it thickens, add the lemon juice or vinegar and salt and pepper to taste. Continue to add more oil until the desired consistency is obtained.

## Marie Rose sauce

2 tbsp mayonnaise

1 tbsp tomato ketchup (organic)

1 tbsp Greek yoghurt (natural)

Mix all the above ingredients together

# Vinaigrette

4 tbsp olive oil
1 tsp mustard
1 tbsp cider vinegar
salt and freshly ground black pepper

Put the salt and vinegar in a bowl and whisk together, add the mustard and continue to whisk, finally add the oil and keep whisking, lastly add the pepper to taste. This can be flavoured with fresh herbs or garlic if desired.

# Caesar salad dressing

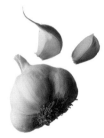

3 cloves garlic
salt and pepper
4 anchovy fillets
1 tsp Worcestershire sauce
2 tsp cider vinegar
4 tbsp olive oil

Crush the garlic and the anchovy fillets together in a bowl with 1 tsp salt and mix. Add the Worcestershire sauce and the vinegar and the freshly ground black pepper and mix together. Slowly drizzle in the olive oil and whisk carefully until the sauce thickens.

# Pesto sauce

2 tbsp pine nuts, very finely chopped
1 large bunch basil leaves, very finely chopped
3 tbsp freshly grated parmesan cheese finely grated
5 tbsp extra virgin olive oil
4 cloves fresh garlic, crushed

Place pine nuts, basil, garlic and cheese into a food processor and process until ground together. With the processor on, slowly pour in the olive oil and continue to process until well blended. Store in a glass jar in the refrigerator.